FLIP THE YOUTH SWITCH

FLIP *the*
YOUTH
SWITCH

Bob Arnot, MD

iBooks

iBooks

Manhanset House
Shelter Island Hts., New York 11965 Tel: 212-427-7139
bricktower@aol.com • www.ibooksinc.com

Library of Congress Cataloging-in-Publication Data
Flip the Youth Switch
Robert Arnot, M.D.
p. cm.
1. Health and Fitness—General 2. Health and Fitness—Longevity
3. Health and Fitness—Healing Fiction, I. Title.

978-1-59687-863-1, Trade Paper

April 2020
Trade Paper
First Printing

CONTENTS

PART III: FIRE: DO GREAT STUFF165

PART IV: THINK BIG TO FEEL GREAT185

APPENDIX: RESOURCES   233

FOREWORD

As this book goes to press, we're in week four of the corona virus lockdown. I've been working 18-hour days, consulting with major medical centers on treatments and risk factors while constructing a course on the virus; supporting hospitals as part of a team scaling up ventilator production. This is a fascinating but grim worldview of whom is at highest risk of a poor outcome. Two key features of surviving COVID 19 emerge which lend themselves tovastly improving our chances of surviving an infection with the virus shouldwe become infected now or in the coming years.They are at the heart of *Flip the Youth Switch*.

IMPROVING BIOLOGICAL AGE.

At a White House, COVID Task Force briefing, Response Coordinator Dr. Deborah Birx was asked about the term "elderly" and the risk it conveyed of a poor outcome. She quickly countered that there are those who are older in chronological age but are biologically younger who may not have the same risk. This lower biological age may be the greatest hedge against severe outcomes from Corona. Older patients on ventilators in London had incredibly poor biological ages, referred to as "black" scores. *Flip the Youth Switch* has the best daily marker of biological age, one that is easy to follow and which improves daily. I've joined a group of 25 and 26-year-olds banding together as Whoop Hardos competing daily to see who has the lowest biological age. A senior Dartmouth professor also views advanced biological age as a marker for the accumulation of chronic illnesses. Those with really a well-managed chronic illness or those who have beaten illness entirely also decrease their risk of a bad outcome.

BATTLE: LOWERING THE RISK OF CHRONIC DISEASE.

Much of aging is the accumulation of chronic illnesses and their deleterious effects. As the chapter BATTLE points out, many of us let ourselves slide into a state of poorer health by not addressing these multiple risk factors. By fiercely battling each and every one of these risks, we also give ourselves the best shot. As Tony Fauci (White House COVID TaskForce, Director of the National Institute of Allergy and Infectious Diseases) articulated, the data show the terrible toll that COVID is taking on our African-American population, with poor access to care for diabetes, high blood pressure, and other illnesses that put these folks at highest risk. Treating chronic illness is incredibly complex and not simply a matter of prescribing a handful of daily medications. BATTLE outlines how. Covid has held some other surprises. In London, younger patients who end up on ventilators had a highBMI(excess body weight in relation to height) or they were smokers. In New York, vapers also ran into trouble.

During this grim time, I hope you find *Flip the Youth Switch* both inspirational to embrace and fun to read. Now is the time to be in the best shape you've ever been in and this is the book to get you there.

—Dr. Bob Arnot

INTRODUCTION

BACK TO THE FUTURE

Fire up the DeLorean, we're going back! With the flip of a switch and a stomp on the accelerator, Michael J. Fox traveled back to the 1950s in an exotic sports car in the film Back to the Future. We're going back too ... back to the days of our youth ... but we're going there as we were then, and we're going to stay! How?

THE LONGEVITY PRIZE

My eyes opened as big as saucers when I first read about the Palo Alto Longevity Prize: $500,000 to reset an aging adult to that of a young one. The foundation had challenged scientists to restore Youth itself. What an idea! Could it be possible? The heart of the quest was embedded in an incredibly powerful marker called "Heart Rate Variability (HRV)," already found on WHOOP and Garmin devices, iPhones, and Apple watches. I began a journey that allowed me to reset my HRV from a 71-year-old to that of a teenager. As you will learn in this book, you can restore youth to the specifications of this ultimate youth prize. Grab a bunch of your friends and you might win the prize itself! A generation of books has promised a decade or so of restoration. The Youth Switch showcases the full restoration of youth using an easily measurable barometer you can track from old to young, watching stunning daily improvements. This journey, too, may be a flip of a switch and a stomp on the gas from old to young!!!

TRANSFORMATION

You'll be dazzled as you experience the metamorphosis from ordinary aging mortal into a lean, young, performance machine. Visualize the transformation of your heart, lungs, and muscle. Feel and perform on a level that's almost beyond imagination with technology-inspired dynamic training programs, far outperforming any conventional training you've tried. Feel the restoration of complete recovery as you flip the switch to youth and see your scores soar with a highly actionable and incredibly easy-to-follow program! Even better, you'll benefit from a daily score you can follow to your greatest success.

THE YOUTH SWITCH

So, what is the Youth Switch? Here's the key background.

Background: We have two nervous systems. The Voluntary Nervous System is the one we are all familiar with. This connects our brain to all the voluntary muscles in our bodies, like biceps, triceps, quads, calves, back, and abdominal muscles; it allows us to climb stairs, write, type, sit, run, throw, walk, jump, bike, etc.

The Autonomic Nervous System: Our bodies also have embedded in them a completely automatic nervous system that you don't have direct control over and are far less aware of. The nerves in the Autonomic Nervous System are connected to organs you don't directly control, such as heart, kidneys, adrenals, intestines, stomach, tear ducts, liver, sweat glands, and blood vessels. How is it controlled? This automatic system reacts to the stimuli your body feeds to it. The switch has two settings. Switch 1 might be turned on by a lion appearing outside your tent or a pedestrian running out in front of your car.

Alternatively, Switch 2 is turned on by a long, restful night's sleep, improved training, quality nutrition, and stress reduction. Let's look closer.

THE YOUTH SWITCH SETTINGS

Switch Setting 1: Fight or Flight is the overdrive that switches on our alertness, pumps out adrenalin, causes heart rate to surge, makes us breathless, and increases sweating, stress hormones, and blood pressure. This response saved early women and men from catastrophe as they fought off predators, ran from wild animals, and advanced into battle. In today's world, we activate this fight-or-flight response for many non-life-threatening events throughout our normal activities, from traffic jams, road rage, and stressful workdays to sitting on hold with customer service or waiting in an interminably long TSA line at the airport. Our emergency response may be turned up all day and well through the night. This extracts a tremendous toll on our bodies. This chronic fight-or-flight stress creates an inflammatory drive. Turning your overdrive on full blast is analogous to aiming a blowtorch at your heart, lungs, muscles, liver, brain, and other internal organs. Yet this is the way most of us live in the 20th century, recklessly and wildly out of balance, careening toward early disaster and hastened aging. Sadly, even in our twenties we have turned up the heat as we ravage our bodies in our quest for success and a wild lifestyle.

Switch Setting 2: Rest and Restore is the second setting of our automatic nervous system. This dampens fight or flight so that we can rest, relax, sleep, fuel, digest, rebuild muscle, and restore our energy, health, and youth. In the Youth Switch, you'll discover that restoration is the biggest and most important part of your day — and highly enjoyable to boot! You'll reset your automatic nervous system to a finely tuned balance that will help you retrieve your lost youth.

THE BALANCED SETTING OF YOUTH

In our youth, our Autonomic Nervous System was balanced with lots of restoration (Switch 2) and occasional pockets of overdrive (Switch 1). With our frenetic modern lifestyles, we move into day-long overdrive, throwing it wildly out of balance and making us sick and old.

Leading researcher Dr. David Mendelowitz studies the Automatic Nervous System at George Washington University.

"Humans are likely born with a good balance of parasympathetic [Switch 2] and sympathetic activity [Switch 1][1] ... But as we get older and face more stress, sympathetic activity increases, putting people at high risk for sudden cardiac death, arrhythmias, high blood pressure, or other cardiovascular diseases," he writes. As this balance erodes with increasing age, we develop a range of diseases from diabetes to hypertension. Dr. Mendelowitz's lab is primarily interested in finding ways to preserve parasympathetic activity (Switch 2). "If you can retain that healthy, subdued heart rate as you get older, that can have many profound health benefits," he said. His team is one of eleven competing for the longevity prize and hoping to restore the balance of parasympathetic and sympathetic activity. The prize committee's vision is that restoring this balance restores youth.

According to Frank M. Longo, Professor and Chair of Neurology and Neurological Sciences at Stanford University, "[T]he timed switch from a functional Autonomic Nervous System to a dysfunctional Autonomic Nervous System may be a key underlying mechanism of chronic diseases and aging."

THE ULTIMATE MEASUREMENT OF YOUTH: HEART RATE VARIABILITY (HRV)

The challenge in awarding such a prize was finding a yardstick that was accurate yet practical enough to measure this restoration of bal-

---

1 http://paloaltoprize.com

ance between sympathetic (Switch 1) and parasympathetic (Switch 2) and ultimately in the restoration of youth on a daily basis. The prize committee selected HRV after careful deliberation as a highly reliable measure of this balance between fight-or-flight and rest-and-restore. We'll learn lots more about HRV in later chapters.

"The $500,000 Homeostatic Capacity Prize will be awarded to the first team to demonstrate that it can restore Homeostatic Capacity (using HRV as the surrogate measure) of an aging reference mammal to that of a young adult," the Palo Alto Prize website states.

To win the prize, Dr. Mendelowitz's team must improve HRV in a test animal — showing that an older mammal can attain the HRV of a younger one. Many research papers have linked a high HRV to good health and low HRV to stress, fatigue, and many cardiovascular diseases. The Autonomic Nervous System regulates HRV and has a range from extremely low for those with constant sympathetic drive to incredibly high for those with high parasympathetic values. Competing teams must show this restoration to a very high HRV, signifying rest and restoration and far less sympathetic stress.

This is a journey I have undertaken, improving my HRV from that of a 71-plus-year-old to that of a 15-year-old in under four months. Have a look at my progress from that of an old man to a young man in his late teens, gauged by HRV. Here's the chart showing my HRV level of an old man — 28 — then peaking at over 100, with averages values in the 70s. This is a journey I will share with you in the Youth Switch.

Clearly, restoring this balance involves incredibly intricate mechanisms at the level of individual cells and even molecules. While HRV is not perfect, in the right setting, it has proven a remarkably reliable marker of this balance that we all want to restore. What's more, it's incredibly easy to measure — just wear a lightweight wristband or press a button on your iPhone. I'm still stunned that I can wake up every morning and see the state of my overall health in a simple measure captured on a wearable device. In fact, my then-6-year-old would grab my iPhone at 7 a.m. to see if dad is going to have a good or bad day!!!

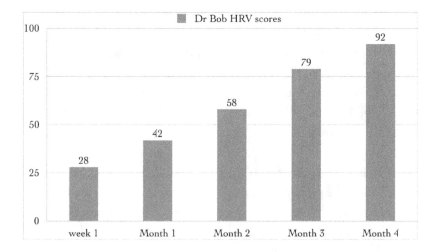

"Healthy longevity depends on preservation of autonomic function, in particular, HRV-parasympathetic function, despite the early age-related decrease,"[2] according to a National Institutes for Health's National Center for Biotechnology publication.

If You Can Measure It, You Can Manage It

Top management experts advise that you can't manage what you can't measure, and that's so true of day-to-day health and fitness. Now, with the advent of new wearable technology, you can measure your daily rest, recovery, fitness, sleep, and strain to counter a low HRV with an incredibly powerful program of enhanced fitness, sleep, and nutrition. HRV forms the core metric. Never before has there been a readily accessible daily measurement of the journey toward youth.

So why would HRV be a good measure of aging? As we have seen, HRV measures the Autonomic Nervous System's setting—whether fight-or-flight or rest-and-restore. Although HRV stands for heart rate variability, HRV has little to do with the heart. The heart just serves as a convenient place to measure the Autonomic Nervous System settings.

2 https://www.ncbi.nlm.nih.gov/pubmed/20381674

Inflamm-aging

Ever had an infected bite on an arm or leg that got out of hand? Redness, swelling, and pain surround the cut as it becomes warm to the touch. Without antibiotics and proper treatment an infection such as this could become overwhelming. Well, this same inflammatory process occurs inside our body unseen. In fact, inflammation is a driving force behind many chronic illnesses, from heart disease to depression, while at the same time decreasing our ability to perform daily activities and increasing our risk of mortality. As we've seen, inflammation is also a prime destructor, causing a progressive loss of function in our vital organs: brain, kidney, heart, liver, muscle. As we age, we develop a low level of inflammation throughout our bodies, which is part of why we feel less well and develop a host of these chronic illnesses. My father used to say that aging is a disease. He was right. Inflammation slowly damages our immune systems, making us more vulnerable to a host of illnesses as it degrades all our major organs. Researchers and doctors can measure the inflammation on the inside with simple blood tests. They are finding a quadrupled increase in the pro-inflammatory substances interleukin [(IL)-6], tumor necrosis factor (TNFα), C-reactive protein (CRP), and serum amyloid A (SAA) in older individuals compared to younger individuals. These increases occur even without chronic illness and are a manifestation of aging itself. Inflamm-aging[3] emerges as a prime driver of aging and represents a highly actionable measurement since it is reflected in HRV rather than these complex cytokine laboratory tests that require your blood be drawn.

The Inflammatory Pathway

With aging, the increased sympathetic drive (Switch1) and subdued rest and recovery pathways (Switch 2) upset the balance in our body and tilt us toward inflamm-aging. The sympathetic pathway

---

3 https://www.ncbi.nlm.nih.gov/pmc/articles/PMC4963991/

stimulates the release of a whole cascade of these pro-inflammatory substances. Think of this imbalance as the primary aging pathway. These changes decrease our bone density, lessen our ability to exercise, lower our mood, decrease our strength, weaken our hearts, and even affect our ability to think. Converging evidence suggests that "… the Autonomic Nervous System (ANS) regulates this inflammatory reflex," reports a recent study.

So, what leads to this inflammation? Stress, fat mass, inflammatory nutrients, and inactivity are the big four. As an example, exaggerated sympathetic nervous system activity associated with low HRV may trigger cardiac arrhythmias and sudden death. Regular exercise/training improves this autonomic balance, as does the ability to truly relax, sleep well, and restore.

Inflamm-aging research: A new meta-analysis of 2,283 studies that appears in the August 2019 issue of the journal Brain, Behavior, and Immunity verifies that a low HRV Switch1 is associated with high inflammation. The paper proposes that "HRV can be used to index activity of the neurophysiological pathway responsible for adaptively regulating inflammatory processes in humans."

So, the challenge has been laid down. Dampen the roar of the inflamm-aging. Bring rest and relaxation into your life for the full restoration of youth. There is, however, an even bigger prize than youth itself: longevity!!!

PART I:

RESETTING THE YOUTH SWITCH

CHAPTER 1

LONGEVITY

"PADDLE, PADDLE, PADDLE! BRACE! BRACE! BREEEEEATHE!!!"

The wind barreled out of the East at 28 knots, pouring down the Kaiwi channel between the Hawaiian Islands of Molokai and Oahu. A jaw-dropping, 20-foot swell crested and broke behind me, hurtling me down a jade-blue, big ocean wave with terrifying speed that was followed by a layer of white froth across its trailing edge. Storm, wind, and ocean swells joined forces to create a fierce washing machine of jagged deep ocean waves. Named the Channel of Bones, the Kaiwi was a horrifying sight to Hawaiian paddlers for millennia and is the world's most dangerous ocean passage.

Surfing and paddling a narrow, unstable, 17-foot stand-up surfboard across the ferocious 32-mile channel, I dug in hard and catapulted the board down wave after wave as my coach yelled, "Paddle, paddle, paddle, rudder right, now rudder left. BRACE, BRACE!!!" This was open-ocean, big-wave, ultra-long-distance surfing at its most challenging — the Molokai 2 Oahu (M2O) World Paddleboard

Championships, called the most difficult waterman's contest on Earth by America's Cup-winning skipper Jimmy Spithill. The Wall Street Journal called M2O one of the four most punishing races of any kind, after you've mastered the ironman. M2O pushes every boundary of human performance to its limits. A heat index of 93 edges the body toward heatstroke as the brain begins to fade. Constant attempts to balance the wildly unstable board bring leg, back, and arm muscles near the verge of uncontrollable, causing vicious and persistent cramping. Your heart hovers around its maximum predicted rate, while your kidneys cease to produce output. The race tests human willpower to its outer fringes. Tendons begin to fray. Joints scream with sharp, searing pain. The stomach twists with discomfort; you are near the threshold of retching. All this is magnified over seven excruciating hours where you fluctuate between the exhilaration of surfing down a giant swell and the fear of death! A crash in the channel three years before dislocated my shoulder, knocked out two teeth, and attracted a shark that chased another competitor out of the race (as observed by Stand Up Paddling [SUP] legend Russ Scully). Several of the world's best athletes dropped out due to injury or heatstroke. In this ultimate test of youth, agility, and virility, with the sport's victors in their late teens and early twenties, I was the oldest person to ever complete the solo race, crossing at the venerable age of 70 and becoming world champion in my age group at both 65 and 70. This is a testament to a program of great training, coaching, and recovery — the ultimate secrets of youth and resetting the youth switch.

Style: Throughout this book, I hope not to appear the least bit immodest in describing my journey. Telling a story through the human body, as do the magnificent documentary Supersize Me and the legendary Younger Next Year, is becoming a fantastic new genre. As a physician and physiologist, I have measured a wide range of physiologic variables in meticulous detail to help you with your own journey, and I hope not in any way to be bragging. I'm just overawed by the results of my journey, and I fervently hope that your journey will become at least as successful. I'm incredibly excited about the success of others, like my 7-year-old in Nordic ski practice or my teammates at the Burlington Surf Club: Spencer Bailey, who followed my paddle steps in the Molokai Race; Laurel Coburn, who crushed it at the Surf to Sound Challenge; and coach Tommy Buday, who performed so well at the World Championships in China. I train with Laurel and Tommy every week in all seasons. I've also been so impressed and heavily influenced by the style of legendary Harvard athlete and WHOOP visionary Will Ahmed in his epic series of podcasts, always so gracious and humble in following the exploits of others. I hope in some small way to emulate his wisdom and style. So, my apologies in advance if I'm a little overeager about my journey. This enthusiasm emanates from a hope that many of you will derive a similar success and joy in a new life of youthful living. I know you can achieve fabulous successes and offer my fondest best wishes on your journey back in time. As you grow older, you'll serve as a tremendous inspiration to others.

TURNING BACK THE CLOCK: BATTLE-TESTED

I wrote Turning Back the Clock twenty-five years ago with a vow to transform myself into a lifelong 25-year-old. This was the grand-daddy of the present rash of books on regaining youth. I was 47 then. I'm 71 now. Did it work? You bet it did, for me and tens of thousands of others, many of whom still follow its advice. That was the vision I created two decades ago and have lived every day since. At age 71, I'm the division winner in the World Championships of Stand Up Paddling and compete in thirty SUP competitions, fourteen cross-country ski races, six ski mountaineering events, and half a dozen gravel grinder bike races each year, including the brutal Race to the Top of Vermont. I'm chief medical officer or on the board of half a dozen humanitarian groups and technology ventures, all while caring for my 7-year-old son Alysdair. I travel the world from displaced persons' health clinics in Iraq and East Africa to ski mountaineering contests in Switzerland and stand-up paddling events in Hawaii.

So how does someone in his eighth decade of life truly become a 25-year-old in spirit, strength, and endurance, and compete in sports designed for teenagers? More importantly, how does a 71-year-old beat the metric established by the Palo Alto foundation for the complete restoration of youth, HRV?

UNIMAGINABLE ADVANCES

"Ladies and gentlemen: The Rolling Stones." My older sons and I watched in astonishment as Mick Jagger exploded onto the stage of the Gillette Stadium with the vigor and energy of a 25-year-old ... at then-age 75. Once unimaginable advances in physical strength and endurance have catapulted a cadre of women and men into true lifelong youth, including the indomitable Mick Jagger. Their inspiring lives demonstrate the astonishing ability to carry vigor, strength, and optimism through middle and into old age while prolonging life itself. These men and women are known as the masters and have spent a lifetime perfecting the art of their chosen sports — in Mick's case, running up to eight miles a day and then dancing and singing for ten miles onstage for each concert. Mick also embodies the antithesis of the rock and rock lifestyle with an abstemious one, eschewing the drugs he once reveled in and embracing tremendous nutrition and restoration. I hope they will inspire you to change course and create a new, hope-filled, and optimistic life of vigor and youth for yourself and your family. You'll find workouts that are astonishingly more effective, and advanced nutrition that will fuel an incredibly satisfying new dimension to your life. If you're currently a Master and have been slowed by injury, overtraining, or age, you'll find fantastic, fresh approaches to revitalize your athletic career and put you back at the top of your game. If you're just beginning, you have an incredible adventure in front of you — and yes, you can catch up.

Americans in their forties, fifties, sixties, seventies, eighties, and nineties are achieving levels of physical prowess long thought impossible. Look at Tom Brady winning his sixth super bowl at age 41. Despite setbacks, Roger Federer was ranked number three in the tennis world at age 38. Dara Torres won three Olympics silver medals in the Beijing Olympics at the age of 41.

And at the end of the spectrum, rigorous scientific studies show an 80-year-old maintaining the fitness of a very fit 35-year-old. During the world cross-country skiing championships this year in Beitostølen, I met an inspiring 96-year-old Russian who still had fire in his eyes and the muscular strength and endurance of the average sedentary 30-year-old There were dozens of competitors in the 80-85 and 85-90-year-old age groups, putting in astonishing performances.

Now you might say, "Easy for you! I'm already suffering the ravages of aging. You have it easy." Not true! Consider this medical history:

Moderate persistent asthma with exacerbations

Severe gastroesophageal reflux

Chronic sinusitis

Complete tear of left and right rotator cuffs

Bilateral hip resurfacing

Aspiration pneumonitis

Mitral valve regurgitation

Severely arthritic knees and ankles

Bronchiectasis

Severely calcified coronary arteries

Four separate arthropathies, including severe osteoarthritis

Sadly, that's me! Yes, staying young becomes a battle. I won't gloss over the difficulties you'll encounter later in life. However, with the right game plan, you can overcome these to restore youth and enjoy an unimaginably great health.

CHAPTER 2

WHAT'S YOUR BLUE-PRINT FOR LIFE?

The peloton ascended out of the mists over the Connecticut River up the steep incline into Lyme, New Hampshire. Twenty-three incredibly fit cyclists accelerated toward the finish line of the Prouty, a 100-mile, highly competitive cancer-fundraising ride. Their jerseys were emblazoned with Dartmouth and US Ski Team logos. Aged 17 to 21, these athletes were among the fastest and fittest in America ... and I was with them! Five decades older, I matched their pace with effortless efficiency. What a dream come true, to perform and feel like an athlete in his early twenties at an age when many Americans were already looking for a rocking chair. For a magic moment in time, as the last wisps of ground fog swept by, I was transported back to my early twenties, when I first arrived on the Dartmouth College campus.

1972: I throttled my Triumph 650 motorcycle's twin-stroke engine, hit the cutoff valve and dropped the kickstand outside of the main administration building at Dartmouth Medical School in Hanover, New Hampshire. I'd landed in paradise. Never had I seen a more idyllic setting, nestled between emerald green foothills, on the outskirts of the legendary White Mountains, and astride the Connecticut River. The campus exuded youth. I arrived with a blueprint for life honed through years of suburban living. I'd finish my workday with a cocktail, enjoy a fine, rare steak dinner with friends, and hang out at the country club on weekends or kick back, watching team sports, fueled with take-out pizza and Miller Lite beer. My physical strength and prowess would slowly fade over the years as I grew a respectable paunch. On retiring at 65, slowly faded while waiting for the grim reaper to strike while I became an increasing burden to my family. Like many Americans, that was the fate I imagined. Popular culture, prime-time sitcoms, and Madison Avenue determined my blueprint for life. As the kickstand struck the ground and the bike came to rest on the pavement in the circular drive, my life changed forever as I discovered a new blueprint for life based on a vigorous physical and adventurous life. At Dartmouth, I learned to cross-country ski race, bound up mountains, row, kayak, run marathons, compete in the Ironman, and travel the globe seeking adventure. From a first-ascent Himalayan climb to volunteering at health clinics in Kenya and Sierra Leone. Famed coach Herman Muchenschnable even invited me to join the legendary Dartmouth Ski Team. At age 22, Dartmouth gave me life's most important gift, one I have treasured to this day: aspirations for a long, vigorous, and youthful life. With this book I hope to help you create a new blueprint for your life, so that you can carry youth, vigor, optimism, and strength into your eighth and ninth decades. Too many of us acquiesce to the lifestyle espoused on daytime talk shows and accept the ever-expanding waistline as the new normal.

Become a Master. Master athletes are the single most successful and fascinating models of "exceptionally successful aging and are the subject of landmark scientific studies by leading physiologists."[4][5] Master athletes strive to maintain and, in some cases, improve upon the performance they have achieved at younger ages with a velocity that accelerates throughout life. Masters are entering sports in droves

---

4 https://www.ncbi.nlm.nih.gov/pmc/articles/PMC2375571/
5 https://physoc.onlinelibrary.wiley.com/doi/full/10.1113/jphysiol.2007.141879

in their forties, fifties, and sixties. They're also breaking records and improving at a rate far higher than younger athletes.

Masters are setting the best new records of any age group. Here are some examples

Marathon: From 1980-2009, running times for ages 70–74 decreased by an incredible 7 percent.[6]

Runners under age 60 did not have a significant improvement in performance in the New York Marathon during the same time period.

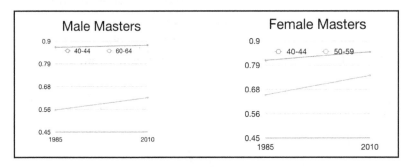

The Master takes an artisanal pride in mastering all of the technical, skill, and training elements of a sport, and continues to compete throughout life, trying to maintain or even improve on his or her performances from a younger age. You can tell them instantly as you look at them. They appear lean and erect, with fierce energy in their eyes. I'd love to inspire you to become a Master athlete. If you are already a Master, you'll find fantastic training, gear, and nutrition knowledge, plus fantastic solutions for aging, sore joints, and muscles that will give you a newfound lease on youth.

THE BLUEPRINT: A NEW TRAJECTORY

Toddler to age 12

Give your children the right "motor" education so that they are ready for a life of fun, fitness, adventure, and robust health. This

6 Lepers and Cattagni, 2012

begins with toddlers through age 12, when you should help them build a large range of motor skills. Children are highly adaptable to mastering a huge inventory of skills. My 7-year-old, Alysdair, skis, plays soccer, cross-country skis, runs, swims, surfs, plays tennis, and climbs mountains.

The key skill development era for kids is from ages 0-12. Just as they learn foreign languages best when young, their nervous systems best adapt to new athletic skills at a young age. These skills will hold for a lifetime, giving them the ability to pick any sport at any stage of life and enjoy it. Yet, even skilled American athletes have become near motor illiterates, socializing in a single sport while failing at many others. Most children are denied a full motor education. Long hours of sitting in the classroom, watching TV, and playing video games have given them tight hip flexors, which prevent them from reaching all the way down to their toes.

We're simply doing a terrible job of teaching our kids youth sports. Sadly, the National Alliance for Youth Sports reports that 70 percent of kids in the United States stop playing organized sports by the age of 13 because "it's just not fun anymore." For most kids, organized sports are a turnoff. Instead, we use the vast majority of youth sports as a screening mill to find star athletes, leaving most kids by the wayside, detesting sports and undertaking a lifelong pathway to a sedentary lifestyle.

Team sports intimidate a large number of children, who shun sport altogether as a result. Then there are the lifelong consequences of concussions and joint injuries. Finally, look at the percentages of young athletes who succeed in college and the pros. Some 2 percent of athletes are given college scholarships. And of those who play NCAA sports, only 2 percent go on to the pros. Specifically, that's 0.9 percent of women's basketball players and 1.5 percent of male football players. There's such a low percentage of success in college and professional sports that I firmly believe we should shift our physical education to giving all children a solid motor literacy in order to open up a lifetime of physical activity, health, and enjoyment to them.

I've always believed we should teach fun life sports from the outset. If you look at the most popular boys' sports, only three of ten could be considered life sports. It's time to shift the focus from using child sports for screening and recruiting to creating major health advantages. I saw this recently with my son's junior soccer team, which I help coach. A few superstar players scored goal after goal and ruled the field, while many of the others just stood on the field and watched. The rest of the players were given no drilling or passing skills. Grade-school sports have become a case of the rich getting richer. Kids who have early success receive all the attention, while most of others just drop out. What we're doing with our team to remedy this is to pick two dribbling drills a week for every child, and then coaching them up to a level where they can be much more confident and competitive.

Don't you want your children to have the broadest exposure to developing skills, with as little pressure as possible?

Here are the components of a motor education, which should be pursued beginning in grade school. The better your child's motor education, the more adaptable he or she will be to a wide range of highly enjoyable sports and pastimes. If you have never had a motor education, this is a great curriculum at any age! Here are some suggestions for your own children and for you to play catch up:

Supervised trampoline (air awareness, body awareness)
Agility ladder
Skipping rope
Coordination drill (Pass ball while on balance board)
Swing on monkey bars (Good for improving timing)
Obstacle course
Soccer drills (YouTube has a ton of these)
Wall climbing (develops full-body awareness)

Here's what I'm doing with my 7-year-old:
Soccer drills before school (We take great foot moves from YouTube and practice one every day)
Tennis (Youth tennis camp on weekends)

Skiing (Mount Mansfield Ski Club training every weekend)
Nordic skiing (Twice-a-week training)
Running (Pre-ski season)
Mountain biking

Ages 13-21:

These are the most important years in developing strong aerobic power. Your heart and lungs respond and adapt quickly to the challenge of running, rowing, cycling, and other aerobic sports. This begins with peak height velocity; that is, the first big growth spurt, around age 12. This is when you want kids to gradually increase the volume of aerobic exercises they undertake. Ages 13-21 are the most effective ages in which to build a robust aerobic engine of fitness and youth — the engine that will carry you into old age as you pursue endurance sports from running and cycling to cross-country skiing, hiking, and SUP. The focus in middle and high school should be on becoming skillful at some wonderful life sport/s and developing a massive aerobic engine. As we'll see, this aerobic power gives you the greatest hedge against aging, and it helps maintain youth many decades longer than most imagine.

The Twenties

In our efforts to recapture our youth, many of us aim to restore ourselves to the shape we were in in our twenties. However, in truth, many millennials are human wrecks. With terrible diets, growing waistlines, and alcohol and substance abuse, there is little to imitate. Many 25-year-olds already exhibit symptoms of the early onset of chronic illnesses, from esophageal reflux disease to diabetes to obesity, heart disease, and serious substance abuse. The disposable income of millennials is dropping due to increases in medical expenses. I'm fitter than almost every 25-year-old I know, and I carry a much greater degree of youth. I routinely beat all 20- and 30-year-olds in long-distance SUP races around New England like the

19.5-mile Blackburn Challenge. Many 20-year-olds see their bodies as a disposable resource, incinerating themselves in pursuit of a career and a good time!

This is the decade to set up great lifetime training, nutrition, sleep, and relaxation habits:

Choose aerobic life sports and acquire the skills to excel

Establish a professional training program

Look at early risk factors that afflict young millennials: binge drinking, obesity, and anxiety

Embrace tremendous nutritional habits

I push my 26-year-old son, Hayden, every day to become fitter, faster, and leaner! Start measuring your HRV daily to both measure your progress and warn of impending doom.

Thirties-Forties

Identify and attack the risk factors that will turn into chronic disease in your fifties and sixties. My 31-year-old, Bobby, has taken up Stand Up Paddling and is a highly accomplished tennis player, but is also learning to address physical ailments early and aggressively. Both 30 and 40 are big birthdays that spur celebrants into wanting to adapt to a rigorous regime of physical activity. Look at the aerobic sports you love and establish a professional training program that will carry you into old age.

Fifties

Age 50 is the biggest of wake-up calls. Friends are already starting to die of heart attacks. The risk factors of your twenties have now matured into full-fledged illnesses. You look with alarm at your spreading midsection, shortness of breath after modest effort, and gray, paunchy face. Begin anew by picking a life sport you truly love. Battle chronic ailments early and effectively. You still have staggering potential to improve your muscles' ability to develop the aerobic engine of youth. Fifty is a great turning point, where you can restore yourself and flip the youth switch back to its original settings from your twenties. It's a time of discovery, where you can choose new sports and activities that are better suited to the next several decades — activities that will safely continue to drive your heart and lung power while maintaining vigorous muscle strength and power. Even if you are reasonably fit, you may have a flawed training program that fails to flip the youth switch and enjoy all the benefits you should.

Sixties-Seventies

Dial it up. Plan to continue improving your aerobic fitness through age 85 and beyond. Be sure you're working out with weights two to three times a week.

In Scandinavia, the most competitive age groups begin at 65. With retirement, men and women finally have the time to devote to a professional training program. When I race in Sweden or Norway, I'm always stunned at how fast the people 65 and over are there.

Eighties

Exceptionally successful aging: An 80-year-old Norwegian grew up on a small farm in a mountainous, roadless region of Norway. "His childhood was dominated by the vigorous manual labor of farm work, fishing, hunting, and berry harvesting, as well as exercise training," the journal Case Reports in Medicine stated, withholding his identity. Each year, he took a seven-day ski trip in the mountains, and he has competed in ultra-endurance ski races in Scandinavia, including the Birkebeiner (54 km) and the Vasaloppet (90 km) ski races. (That's one of my favorites!) He also competed in the Birkebeiner mountain bike race (89 km) and the Birkebeiner mountain half marathon (21 km). Did it pay off?

The Cornerstone of youth: heart and lung power: The Department of Cardiology, St. Olav's University Hospital, Trondheim,

Norway, conducted a key test called maximum oxygen uptake (VO2 max) on the Norwegian. In this book, VO2 max is the most important scientific term you will learn and is the cornerstone of youth. VO2 max is a global performance measurement that combines your heart's ability to pump blood and your lungs' ability to deliver oxygen to exercising muscle. VO2 max predicts your longevity and defines your fitness age, which could be decades younger ... or older ... than the age on your driver's license.

The Norwegian man scored a VO2 max of 50 mg/kg. This is the equivalent of a superior score for a very fit and active 35-year-old Norwegian man or an inactive 25-year-old Norwegian. The average 80-year-old scores only a 22. To put this further into perspective, an Olympic Canoeing Gold Medalist has a VO2 max of only 48. This placed this Norwegian in a position to compete and win a race against a 35-year-old, given all the fitness, skill, and athletic prowess developed over a lifetime. His maximum heart rate was a stunning 175 beats per minute. He had 49 percent muscle with lean and superb lung function. Dazzling!!! He lived the dream of lifelong youth, the most fantastic goal of mankind for millennia.

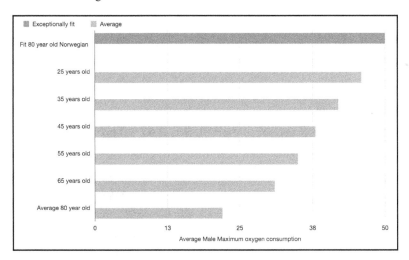

Nineties

Never too late to start: The "Amazing Mavis" Lindgren was a worldwide phenomenon. This formerly overweight nurse embarked

on a marathon career in her seventies after starting a walking program. She set the world marathon record for her age in Napa Valley at 4:34 at age 80. In her career, she ran seventy-five marathons and had an extremely high quality of life. She earned the nickname "amazing" after winning gold and silver in the World Master's games with stage four cancer. Her case study, as reported on the website Diabetes Diet Dialogue, concluded: "It is never too late to start exercising and, an unusually high VO2 max is possible even in old age." She completed the San Diego Marathon in 7:07 at aged 91!!! Her VO2 max at 75 was a stunning 39, the equivalent of a sedentary college-aged woman.

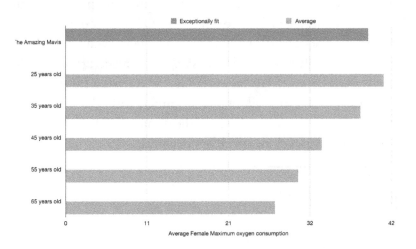

MEDIOCRE GOALS VERSUS GOALS THAT INSPIRE

One reason so few of us pursue a program to transform ourselves is that the goals are too modest. We're also not so sure that becoming 50 at 70 or 40 at 60 is much of a goal. The core goal of this book is to show that you can reconstitute youth, flipping the youth switch from old to young. This is a new, novel, and inspiring goal, but one that you may achieve, given daily metrics to follow your progress.

As my friend Dean Ornish discovered, people will reach for fantastic goals even if they don't appear achievable rather than reaching for mediocre ones. Why? Because they may feel no improvement after achieving a mediocre goal. However, with outrageous goals, participants feel so fantastically better that they stick with the program. Dean has demonstrated the reversal of coronary artery disease over five years of diet, exercise, and stress reduction. He found that big changes motivated people. For years the public health community has pandered to the American public, encouraging small steps even as we have grown more and more obese and have witnessed a catastrophic increase in diabetes. Clearly, pandering doesn't work, as evidenced by the dramatic increases in obesity, heart disease, and diabetes. People will work hard for noble goals. That's why I'm asking you to reach for the sky and aim for recreating youth!

In this book we'll focus on five key steps:

1. Stimulus: First is the remarkable increase in life expectancy that the devoted Master athlete attains with a scientifically developed training program that can yield as much as a 40 percent decrease in all-cause mortality. This is much easier than most athletes realize; you simply strip away all of the coaching jargon and focus on improving your oxygen delivery system.

2. Fuel: Second is the effect of incredibly powerful nutrients. We'll focus on a high polyphenol intake, associated with a 30 percent decrease in all-cause mortality. These percentage decreases in all-cause mortality are staggering There is no medication or medical treatment available that can come anywhere close to these breathtaking decreases. We'll also look at the special proteins needed to grow bigger, stronger muscles and the fuels that make exercise a joy.

3. Fire: Do great stuff! You'll wake up with limitless energy and startling mental clarity, and you'll gain the motivation to keep it up if you have a lifelong mission to inspire others.

4. Think BIG to feel GREAT: A rich portfolio of learning and professional activities deliver the motivation and mental energy to maintain lifelong vigor.

5. Battle: Finally, we have the battle against the chronic illnesses that whittle away at our reserves and slowly extinguishes our youth.

CHAPTER 3

STIMULUS AND RECOVERY

The missing ingredients: Why do so many older people wither while others like these spectacular athletes thrive? The reason is summed up in one word: stimulus. On the basis of rigorous scientific study, the US National Library of Medicine reported that researchers conclude the ability to maintain a high training stimulus with advancing age is "... emerging as the single most important means of limiting the rate of decline."

The human body requires enough intensity to stay young. The wildly successful Master can still undertake the amount and intensity of exercise in each workout necessary to maintain youthful performance into old age.[7] Stimulus is the true fountain of youth, what Ponce de Leon sought half a millennium ago, yet the concept of stimulus is unknown to all but a small group of research scientists.

WHY WE FAIL

Most of us just can't apply the right amount of stimulus because we are too stiff, sore, over-trained, unmotivated, in a sport that

---

7 https://physoc.onlinelibrary.wiley.com/doi/full/10.1113/jphysiol.2007.141879

no longer delivers for us, or just in the wrong training program. Examples are:

Groundhog-day-itis — a routine fitness buff who just gets slower and stiffer through a monotonous training program that doesn't vary from day to day

The fitness buff who eschewed technology and sports science and is lost in training programs left over from high school

A tennis player with arthritic knees who can no longer sprint to the net for the hours required to be fit

A runner whose recurrent overuse injuries stand in the way of a reliable training program, and who has curtailed total mileage and intensity

A squash player whose back limits intensive play

A swimmer with debilitating shoulder injuries whose pace has slackened

An iron athlete with hip arthritis

A walker who develops plantar fasciitis

A cyclist whose arthritis extends to both kneecaps, limiting intensity and volume

The former athlete who has just surrendered to time and waits for Father Time to catch up

The sedentary individual who just never knew the tremendous benefits of intense exercise.

This book will give you the sports, activities, professional training programs, and other solutions needed to apply the stimulus that keeps you young. As you'll read, the right stimulus targets youth with extreme specificity, is easily incorporated into any training program, and requires far less time than you would imagine.

Research shows the tremendous effect that exercise can have on damping the inflammation that makes us sick and accelerates aging. However, this program embodies a very specific prescription of duration, frequency, and intensity. These three elements drive the increase in VO2 max that is so vital to youth and longevity. These are only possible, though, by achieving strong recoveries with lots of rest and great sleep that makes such workouts possible, as we will see in great detail.

DEVELOP A SMART TAKE ON EXERCISE SCIENCE

As a lifelong student of exercise science, I've long held that physiology, motor learning, and biomechanics are among the most interesting intellectual pursuits. A solid foundation in these subjects will make you a superior athlete and deliver unimaginable dimensions to your fitness. What upsets me is how many really smart people take great care in understanding the finest nuance of their finances, vacations, and careers, but ruthlessly dumb down fitness — making their workouts exceedingly dull and unproductive. They mock me for wearing my WHOOP and Garmin watches, for taping tech gear to my SUP board ... until I pass them in a race! These devices teach you so much more and make your exercise and its benefits far more precise and enjoyable. Yet, so many smart people are utterly dismissive of any sophistication in their exercise or fitness. This is probably a throwback to the day when phys ed was considered the lowest end and dumbest of the classes we took in high school. These Luddites think there is something immoral or unethical in making exercise any more complex than a walk in the park! By dismissing sophistication in training, they miss a staggering opportunity to dramatically improve their fitness, how they feel, and their biological age. I meet so many men and women in their forties, fifties, and sixties who work out but just don't look fit. They've lost a huge amount of their potential, surrendering muscle and fitness to ignorance! I get the biggest kick out of looking at photos of experts on aging, few of whom look like they take their own advice!

Should you run into this resistance from friends you are trying to encourage to try new technology, I got this advice from WHOOP founder and CEO Will Ahmed: "Ask doubters, 'Have you ever overtrained or had a less than desirable performance?' If you think sleep and recovery are important to you, you must measure them to manage them. You may say you can FEEL whether you have recovered and are ready for a big workout, but feelings tend to be chest up," Will said. "You could have a head cold and a great performance. Feelings are pretty overrated. You cannot feel slow-wave or REM sleep. Physiologic indicators allow you to find a flow state with unbelievable performance where everything feels easy."

Unlocking the secrets of exercise science allows youth to become a true Master.

Here are the four basic areas embedded in this book:

1. Physiology
2. Nutrition
3. Biomechanics
4. Motor learning

Knowing these subjects will gain you more years of life and far more life in those years, making this the best investment you can make. Most athletes are not born. You can become a GREAT athlete and add immeasurable enjoyment and success to life by using these principles. Olympians do, and they bring home gold. Some may be no more capable than you; they've just received and applied a far better exercise science education. Many athletes just run, walk or hike. Yet, there are spectacular added dimensions to your enjoyment and ability to flip the youth switch by mastering complex sports like Skimo and SUP.

Foremost is exercise physiology and understanding the concept of maximum oxygen uptake. This may appear a bit complex, but I've broken it down into small, digestible pieces. You'll love learning about VO2 max, the heart of youth. The vast majority of us with regular workouts never learn to improve VO2 max. As you do, you'll make tremendous gains.

THE ENGINE OF YOUTH

A large and sustained oxygen demand lies at the heart of recreating youth. That means activating the largest groups of muscles to create the most sustained and powerful oxygen demand. The data and analytics platform on a large WHOOP database captured millions of hours of training. (WHOOP is a membership-based fitness program that measures both individual and team statistics electronically to enhance performance.) The WHOOP data demonstrate that aerobic athletes recorded higher HRV scores than all other athletes. So, for example, cross-country skiers, employing every major muscle group in the body for hours-long races, tax the heart and lung systems to their maximum. Many athletes wonder if cross-training, racket sports, or weight training might provide a similar stimulus. While these are great activities and provide a good stimulus, they do not create the tremendous stimulus of a large aerobic load. That's why I emphasize choosing endurance sports that require the highest oxygen demand. Now sure, you cross-train within that framework, doing a day or two in the gym or playing tennis or squash. However, it is the singular focus on precise aerobic development that delivers the very highest quality results. Only by taxing precisely the same muscles over and over again do the new blood vessels and mitochondria grow to their greatest potential and deliver the best results. There's tremendous satisfaction in watching your training intensity and volume increase year after year. Athletes literally improve from their mid-fifties into their eighties. Developing a large MVO2 (myocardial oxygen consumption) and delivering a large aerobic training stimulus through a dynamic training program forms the central thesis of this book. Let's take a closer look.

VO2 MAX: THE ULTIMATE BAROMETER OF YOUTH AND LONGEVITY

A large VO2 max is the ultimate barometer of longevity and the most fantastic hedge against aging. Those individuals scoring the very highest VO2 max[8] have:

---

8 https://www.topendsports.com/testing/records/vo2max.htm

Youngest fitness age

Lowest risk of heart disease

Biggest reserve against aging

Greatest longevity

Lowest risk of all-cause mortality

Unparalleled potential at success in endurance sports

The American Heart Association (AHA) reports that a low VO2 max is associated with increased risk of cardiovascular disease and all-cause mortality. According to the AHA:

"People who have lower cardiorespiratory fitness also have higher risk of developing certain cancers, including lung, breast, and gastrointestinal cancers."

"VO2 max can predict risk of early death even better than some traditional risk factors like being overweight, high cholesterol, or smoking. So, you could say fitness age might be a better predictor of longevity than chronological age."

The great news is that VO2 max can be greatly improved whether you're in your teens or your seventies. Athletes have venerated a large VO2 max for generations, yet the concepts behind the number remain shrouded in mystery. I recall so clearly being stunned by the lean, raw athletic prowess of the US rowing team as they exited the Connecticut River into the Dartmouth boathouse in 1972. They appeared as a different species! I overheard them comparing VO2 max scores like baseball players would batting averages — with great reverence and adulation. So, let's lift the veil and look under the hood at VO2 max to give you a fantastic vision of how much there is to improve!

Overview: VO2 max has two major components, the supply side and the demand side. The supply side is the pump, comprised of heart, lung, arteries, and blood. This heart-and-lung system delivers oxygen and fuel to exercising muscle. The demand side is the muscle itself, which consumes oxygen and fuel to create energy. Let's look at each component individually, since tremendous improvements can be made in each of them. Just as a car can be made faster with a bigger engine, better tires, more robust racing transmission, and air scoops, the human body has a fantastic variety of parts that all lend themselves to more speed, power, endurance, energy ... and youth.

1. The Pump

Increased blood volume: The first and fastest change in response to training is the increase in the amount of blood circulating in your body.

Your blood volume will increase from 2.8 liters to 3.3 liters in just two weeks. This increased volume supercharges your heart by jamming more blood into it. This begins improving your VO2 max.

More red blood cells: Exercise stimulates your bone marrow to produce many more red blood cells, so you can carry more oxygen to your muscles. Training at altitude also increases red blood cell production, making altitude a favored type of training for competitive athletes and Olympians.

Bigger pump: As you adapt to exercise, the increased volume of blood overfills your heart's pumping chambers and stretches them, so there is more blood to pump out with each beat. Over time, the heart further adapts by growing a larger main pumping chamber and stronger, more dynamic, and powerful muscle. Doctors observe an increased size of the left ventricle on X-ray, EKG, and echocardiogram, and they term this an athlete's heart. In a comparison of runners, cyclists, and track athletes, the cyclists had by far the largest ventricular volume and wall thickness, due to the tremendous amounts of blood they circulate over the many hours they compete. The famed Tour de France course often measures over 100 miles a day.

Slowed heart rate: During training, your heart will begin to beat more slowly at any given pace. So, you might have noted 96 beats per minute while walking a fourteen-minute mile. After training, you might find it beats 88 times per minute at the same pace. This allows the heart more time to fill more fully, so that the left ventricle is jammed even fuller with blood before pumping. This is a readjustment of your fight-or-flight sympathetic nervous system, so you'll start to feel far more relaxed throughout your day. You'll see much lower resting heart rate on WHOOP, Garmin, and other wearables. A low resting heart rate is a hallmark of elite athletes.

Mine beats 42 times a minute versus an average of 60 plus beats a minute for the untrained; the latter is cited as normal by the American Heart Association and the Mayo Clinic.[9]

Increased stroke volume: The total amount of blood pumped during a single contraction of the heart is termed stroke volume.

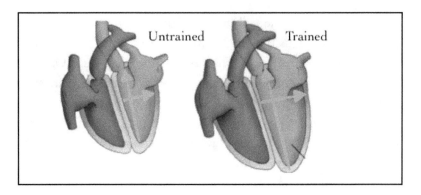

An intensive, six-month training program causes a substantial increase in stroke volume. Let's have a look:

Untrained athlete: 100 ml/beat
Trained athlete: 150 ml/beat
Highly trained 220+ ml/beat

How much training does it take? An intensive, four-day-a-week, one-hour-a-day program at up to 90 percent VO2 max resulted in a 23 percent increase in ejection fraction (the percentage of blood that is pumped out of the heart's ventricles with each contraction).

Easier blood flow: Stroke volume also increases because the heart meets far less resistance when the main aortic valve opens and pumps blood into the body's main arteries. This allows the ventricle to empty more fully. Think of a garden hose with a nozzle. When

9 https://biostrap.com/blog/resting-heart-rate-70-is-the-new-90/

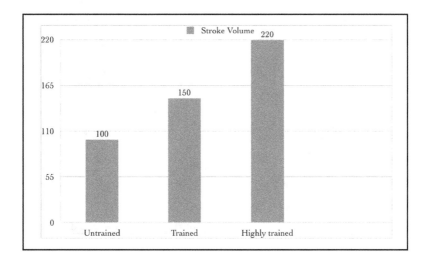

twisted down so there is a very fine and powerful stream, there is tremendous resistance, and you'll have to turn up the faucet to get enough water pressure. But if you untwist the nozzle, the water flows out much more easily. This is a very important training effect, as your entire vascular system decreases resistance with training — which is a terrific health consequence.

Breathing deeper and faster: As you exercise at higher intensities, breathing harder is the first observation you will make. Breathing deeper and faster puts more oxygen into the red blood cells More blood flows into the right side or your heart, which supplies the lungs, to match the increase in breathing. Here's what the maximum breathing looks like:

100 L/minute untrained
150 L/minute trained
200 L/minute well-trained

The biggest adaptation in your lungs to exercise is to use much more of the upper parts of the lung to load up red blood cells with oxygen.

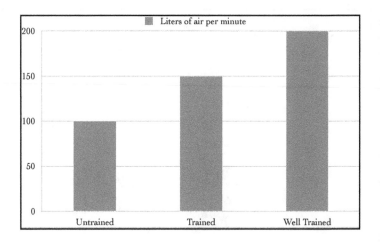

2. The Factory

So, let's take a break. We've looked at improvements with training. These are called "central," or supply-side, adaptations in your heart, lung, arteries, and blood vessels. We've seen that more blood supercharges the heart, which pumps more blood more freely, while more of the lung loads oxygen into more red blood cells. Younger athletes will have huge improvements in these central adaptations. Now let's focus in on the exercising muscle itself, where most athletes will enjoy tremendous successes. Here's what happens in and around muscle with a good dose of aerobic training.

More small blood vessels: Capillaries are the microscopic blood vessels that encircle muscle cells to deliver fuel and oxygen. With training, the number of capillaries dramatically increases to deliver these essential elements of energy production for exercise. Imagine an interstate road network in the middle of Montana, with few secondary roads. Now picture that interstate network around New York City, with thousands of extra miles of feeder roads, secondary routes, and residential neighborhoods. The latter can deliver millions more packages a day than can the Montana network.

You will greatly increase the number of capillaries to increase delivery to the specific muscles you are training. Each muscle fiber you train will have a greatly enhanced number of capillaries. Exercise also recruits more of the existing capillaries and shifts blood flow to the muscles working hardest and away from less active tissues in the body. This increased number of capillaries is one of the most important improvements in VO2 max, and this can occur at any age in life. Blood also becomes less sticky, so it flows more smoothly through these microscopic blood vessels. Training is highly specific, so you'll want the same activity to develop the most blood vessels in the specific muscle you are using. You'll want at least four days a week devoted to one specific aerobic activity to develop specific capillaries. Cross-training and other sports are fine on your recovery days.

Increased oxygen storage: Myoglobin is the molecule used to store oxygen inside of muscle cells. Myoglobin facilitates the shuttle of oxygen to the energy-producing factories inside. Think of myoglobin molecules as the warehouses with raw materials ready to be fed into nearby factories. Endurance muscles develop tremendous amounts of myoglobin, giving them their characteristic reddish color and the ability to store much more oxygen right inside the muscle cell for easy access during exercise.

Bigger and more numerous energy factories: Mitochondria are the heart of the body's energy production system. These fantastic little factories contain a production assembly line, importing oxygen and fuel to create massive amounts of energy. With training, mitochondria increase in number and size to become far more robust and powerful. Example: The number of mitochondria in trained rats increased 15 percent in twenty-seven weeks, and mitochondrial size increased a whopping 35 percent!!!

The overall volume of training has the most pronounced effect on the increased number and size of mitochondria — and fantastic improvements can still be achieved late in life.

Youth at Its Core

Mitochondria are youth. With aging, the mitochondrion's capacity to generate energy fades. More than any other goal in this book, it is the mitochondrion that you want to multiply, grow, and increase, in energy-producing power. The secret, as you will see in the training programs below, is high-intensity training. You'll find two kinds — the five-minute internal that develops VO2 max best, and the short interval, such as HIIT (high-intensity interval training), which may have its greatest effect on the mitochondrion. So effective is intense exercise that research shows high-intensity cycling reversed the age-related decline in mitochondrial function.

A Mayo Clinic study showed that young volunteers increased their mitochondrial capacity by 49 percent with intensive exercise. However, an older group in the study had a stunning 69 percent increase.

Like any factory, mitochondria spew out toxic substances called free radicals. Countering these with a strong nutritional program is a vital part of staying young and preventing damage. The "Fuel" section of this book has a complete program that harnesses the power of polyphenols to dampen inflammation and oxidation.

Raw chemical power: Power itself is embodied in the chemical reactions that transform fuel into energy within the mitochondrion. These reactions are driven by enzymes that speed these chemical reactions up enormously. Scientists measure the amounts of these enzymes in response to exercise to gauge the effectiveness of training. One of the enzymes is called SDH (succinate dehydrogenase). Jogging just twenty minutes a day increases SDH by 25 percent. This enzyme activity diminishes with aging, which may be a big part of why we get old and feel old. You'll discover that it is vital to keep these enzymes at the highest levels possible! These enzymes increase substantially over seven months of training.

Measuring muscle oxygen consumption: I have made improving mitochondria the heart of my training program with fantastic success, since this is where the greatest improvements can be attained. The biggest breakthrough is a new piece of exercise gear that allows you to directly measure the oxygen consumption of mito-chondria while you work out. (Two companies, Humon and Moxy, manufacture these body oxygenation measurement systems.) I use one of these devices every day in training. I push as hard as possible to drive the oxygen consumption readings from green to orange to deeply into the red, knowing the red reading is the maximum intensity interval with the most fantastic training effect. We'll look at this more in the equipment section, but in my view, muscle oxygen consumption, or $SmO2$, is the single most important value you can measure during exercise, replacing heart rate and other lesser measures. As you get better, you'll go far faster and harder before you hit a red.

WHAT TO EXPECT

As an athlete over forty, you'll make solid but limited gains in your heart and lung capacity. However, the mitochondria have a phenomenal upside and will respond to intense training into your nineties, keeping you young and incredibly energetic. Remember, these fantastic little energy factories are energy. There are 2,000 mitochondria per muscle cell and 5,000 in heart muscle, which is the most active muscle in the body. Mitochondria even have their own DNA, and when they are dysfunctional, a long list of illnesses and aging itself result.

Summary: OK, Let's put this all together. First, let's look at an untrained individual trying to work out, then at a fully trained Master.

Novice: Say you start walking up a steep hill at a fast pace. You'll first notice how hard, even labored, your breathing is. Your muscles are creating a tremendous demand for oxygen, but your heart and lungs can't deliver enough. There just aren't enough blood vessels to deliver the oxygen you need, and there are too few energy-producing factories to produce energy. In a moment of panic, the muscle cells switch over to making energy without oxygen. The by-product is lactic acid. Your muscles start to burn, get tight, and feel fatigued. You're breathing even harder, possibly gasping for a breath. You slow in pain and defeat, sure that an ambitious exercise program is just not for you. Even if you are a trained athlete trying a new sport or coming back after a long break, you'll have similar feelings. This discourages many from training. On my muscle oxygen devices, a beginner will go from green to orange to red in as little as fifteen seconds, showing very little capacity for delivering oxygen. You'll be stunned at how quickly our fortunes reverse with a well-thought-out, professional training program. These hills will soon become effortless, and you will seek bigger challenges. Just ease into them!

The fitness enthusiast: If you make an effort several days a week to jog or work out in the gym but find you're not getting results or are slowing down and feeling the effects of aging, you'll derive enormous success by embracing the dynamic training and recovery programs in this book, improving your MVO2 and driving your HRV to new highs.

The Master: As a lifelong endurance athlete, you've maximized your heart and lung adaptations years ago. Your biggest upside is in training muscle. You can expect to build many more capillaries around your muscles' cells, increase the size of your mitochondria, and massively increase the chemical enzymes inside that produce energy. Since you are increasing oxygen demand, your VO2 max will increase substantially more because of these muscle adaptations than your heart and lungs. The key for a Master is delivering this large aerobic stimulus in training. This may mean a change in sport to lower the load on your joints and increase oxygen demand.

SUCCESS

Now let's fast-forward a few months. You head up the same hill at a stiff pace. Your muscles demand energy, and the energy factories gear up to meet the demand. With much enhanced capacity, mitochondria start spewing out an enormous amount of energy. Your muscles quickly signal your heart and lungs for more oxygen. Your heart is now loaded with a huge amount of blood, which primes the left ventricle. Your stroke volume increases to meet demand. Your lungs use their entire capacity to pack more oxygen into a vastly increased number of blood cells. With tremendous ease, your heart unloads its supply of blood into the heart's main arteries, which accept the new load of blood with little resistance. As the blood arrives at the muscle, there is a vast new network of blood vessels to accept the oxygen, then transfer that oxygen into cells and into greatly increased and improved energy producing factories. You're not only exercising with ease, but your body feels great. There's no strain, no pain, and no gasping or acute shortness of breath. Now exercise has become a joy, as you can do more and more at higher and higher tempo with nothing but positive feedback. You're also delivering a tremendous aerobic stimulus and will start to get amazing recovery stores, feeling far more relaxed and confident. The bigger the aerobic stimulus, the better your recoveries and higher your HRV will soar on rest days. So, since the largest aerobic stimulus wins, let's look at which athletes achieve the highest VO2 max.

CHAPTER 4

VO2 MAX

Who scores highest? Who are the biggest winners of all? Here are the highest recorded VO2 max scores. The scale goes from a low of 17 to an all-time record high of 97.5. Athletes recite their VO2 max with great pride, as a badge of distinction.

Men

97.5: Cyclist Oskar Svendsen

96.0: Cross-country skier Espen Harald Bjerke

92.0 Ultra-endurance mountain and ski mountaineering racer Kílian Jornet Burgada (I'm a huge Kíllian fan. He's climbed 27,000 feet in a day and is the ultimate sky runner. He also does a form of cross-country skiing called ski mountaineering racing, or Skimo, that requires first racing up the mountain before racing down.)

92.0 Pikes Peak Marathon record holder Matt Carpenter

81.0 Track and fielder Jim Ryun (last American to hold the world record in the mile run)

80.9 Norwegian soccer player Øyvind Leonhardsen

Women

78.5 Distance runner Joan Benoit Samuelson
76.6 Cross-country skier Bente Skari
76.0 Cyclist Flávia Oliveira

In carefully selecting a life sport, consider the sports and activities that build the very biggest reserve over a lifetime. As you can see, cyclists, Nordic skiers, and hill runners do the very best of all. While VO2 max can be directly measured and your fitness age accurately determined, this book's appendix has a variety of self-tests.

Running, cycling, and Nordic skiing register the highest VO2 max scores for women as well. However, women have lower measured VO2 max than men. The questions are whether there are just fewer women in these sports and therefore a narrower selection, or whether even more talented women go into high-skill sports, leaving fewer women in the pool of these key aerobic sports.

LONGEVITY

Arguably, the most objective measurement of an elite athlete's ultimate success is longevity.[10] Scientists calculate longevity based on the statistical calculation of mortality matched to your demographics and risks. Mortality is the measure researchers, epidemiologists, pharmaceutical companies, and disease-tracking physicians use in following large populations of people. The specific measure is called "all-cause mortality," and it includes any cause of death, from accidents to cancer to diabetes to heart disease, etc. There are enormously significant studies, such as Harvard's healthcare professional studies, that assess risk factors that may lead to death. These may include cigarette smoking, ultraviolet light exposure, poor diet, and lack of exercise among many others. The Harvard study also looks at specific interventions, such as lycopene, calcium, fatty acids, and

---

10 https://www.ncbi.nlm.nih.gov/pmc/articles/PMC4534511/

diet. Clinical trials test the measurement of specific interventions, for example, new cancer drugs.

Here are other examples of all-cause mortality measurements:

Populations: e.g., Native Americans

Disease groups: e.g., diabetes

Diets: e.g., the Mediterranean diet

Beverages: e.g., coffee, tea, red wine

Dietary ingredients: e.g., polyphenols

So, who lives longest? Athletes!!! There are substantial decreases in all-cause mortality seen in groups of athletes. Tour de France cyclists are among the most long-lived, averaging eight years longer than the general population. Thirteen percent of Olympic medalists were alive thirty years after their Olympic success than their non-Olympic peers. And even leisure time activity increases life expectancy by 4.7 years.

HEALTHY LIFE EXPECTANCY

"Healthy Life Expectancy" is the measure of the number of years you may expect to live in good health. In West Virginia it's just 63.8 years, according to the Centers for Disease Control. So, if you're 54, you have just ten good years left on average. Pretty frightening. Even if you live in the top ranked state, Minnesota, your health life expectancy is only 70.3 years. That's just five good years after the conventional retirement age. For many people, living past their healthy life expectancy just isn't much fun, as they battle a range of chronic illnesses in pain and great discomfort. Winston Churchill may be the best example, rumored to have said he "... died at 50 but took another forty years to lie down." Churchill drank, smoked cigarettes, and enjoyed fabulous cuisines but suffered tremendously from a variety of chronic ailments — even suffering a stroke as prime minister. Ultimately, you want to live young as long as you possibly can — in the best possible health.

CHAPTER 5

BUILDING A LARGE VO2 MAX

Every endurance athlete craves a large VO2 max. You will too! Nothing translates into living a long and better life than a robust VO2 max. Here are the most important principles in building yours!

You'll experience one of the remarkable feelings in training and fitness. As your muscles gradually demand more and more oxygen, they will drive your lungs into long, deep respirations that inspire a deep sense of calm and restoration. Although many yoga exercises try to mimic the deep breathing of a fully aerobic workout, none come close to the sense of satisfaction and fulfillment that arrives with true deep breathing driven by physiological necessity.

For most big muscle groups, VO2 max is ultimately about having muscles pull oxygen from the bloodstream, so the more muscles you work hard, the higher the oxygen demand.

Choose sports with the biggest muscle groups, like hill bounding, cross-country skiing, stand up paddling, ski-mountaineering racing, cycling, running, and rowing:

Low impact: The destructive forces of exercise have ruined a generation of knees and hips and created a billion-dollar joint replacement industry. The ability to exercise over a lifetime is severely curtailed by high-impact activities. Sports with a very low impact allow for large volumes of exercise without injury or overuse. You can see the huge impact on the knee in golf, tennis, jogging, and stair-stepping. By contrast, rowing, training on ellipticals, and tread-mill-walking put a very low load on your joints.

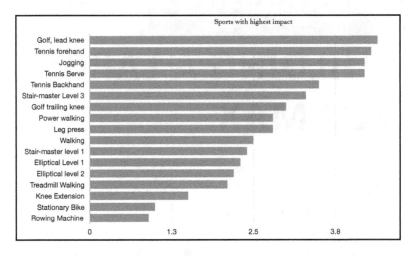

Large volume: Low-impact load allows an enormous training volume. I've competed in a 100-mile cross-country ski race, an 86-kilometer, one-day Nordic ski race, and many 52-kilometer paddleboard races with far less exhaustion than running a marathon. I couldn't possibly run or walk that far, especially on a daily basis. However, I could ride 50–100 miles a day, ski 20–30 kilometers a day, or paddle thirty-five miles a day for weeks. Choosing activities like cycling, stand-up paddling, Nordic skiing, hiking, or hill bounding allows you to safely undertake big training volumes.

High stimulus: Intervals allow a huge training load to be put on the body and are ultimately responsible for building heart and lung volume, neuromuscular coordination, strength, and speed. You can apply a tremendous stimulus with hill bounding, cycling, Nordic skiing, and SUP, leveraging large muscle groups to deliver a huge stimulus with little pain or perceived exertion. The key is finding the very best way for you to leverage your major muscle groups. High stimulus requires a large background of longer, slower distances to build up your body to withstand the stresses of that high stimulus.

Elasticity: With aging, muscle elasticity is lost. The shock absorbers in your muscles are less effective and the pounding of running or walking goes more directly into the joints, tendons, and ligaments, increasing the risk of overuse, injury, and arthritis.[11] The best youth sports make up for this loss of springiness. Some, like cycling, restore elasticity. I love the expression, "Put some bounce back into your step." Put springiness back into tendons, ligaments, and the connective tissue within muscles:

Avoid sports that put high load on your joints.

Use equipment that absorbs the shock and impact of working out, like bicycles.

Try sports that build elasticity by preloading muscles, such as cycling and SUP.

Undertake dynamic stretching.[12]

Yoga actively stretches muscles far more than routine stretching programs.

Rumble foam rollers dig into the supporting tissue of muscle to loosen them up so you can stretch more dynamically.

Avoid overuse: Will your sport result in frequent overuse injuries, limiting your ability to get the volume and intensity you need to stay young? We'll recommend sports with the lowest risk.

Find your sweet spot. One of the greatest secrets of training is the exact exercise prescription necessary to increase VO2 max. This is a three- to five-minute time period of intense exercise. This stimulates the entire oxygen transport system to its maximum and achieves the ultimate training effect. This once-a week-training is the heart of increasing your VO2 max.

11 https://www.ncbi.nlm.nih.gov/pubmed/28647869
12 http://www.stretchstationsd.com/blog/improve-muscle-elasticity/

BEST SPORTS FOR A LARGE VO2 MAX

So now let's look at which sports deliver the highest VO2 max and what their advantages are to you. I've included some practical examples, since fewer of you have access to Nordic skiing or rowing.

Cycling

Cycling may seem like an outlier, since cycling uses a smaller group of muscles than rowing or Nordic skiing. However, cycling leverages the body's biomechanics, creating tremendous amounts of power for prolonged periods of time with low perceived exertion. Also, as a cyclist gets out of his seat and climbs, all the major muscle groups are engaged, as they are in mountain biking.

Scientists studying triathlons compared running, swimming, and cycling. They found that cyclists had the least age-related decline in performance.[13] Why? They concluded that age-related decline in endurance sports depends on the kind of "locomotion." The bike is one of the finest technical instruments for making the body far more mechanically efficient. The key is keeping a high cadence so that you are taking stress off your knees as you develop power, endurance, and elasticity in your main quadricep muscles.

Here are several reasons why cycling delivers such a significant training stimulus:

Cycling is the most mechanically efficient, allowing for huge power settings but at a very high cadence, so the load on the muscle is far less

Cyclists are capable of a much greater volume of training, at both endurance pace and at high intensity (I've competed in a 500-mile. 24-hour race in Central Park).

There are fewer injuries due to too much of this type of exercise.[14]

Cyclists can train for longer periods of time before fatigue sets in.

Cyclists can train at a much higher threshold before starting to make

---

13 Bernard et al., 2010; Lepers et al., 2010, 2016; Lepers and Stapley, 2011
14 Easthope et al., 2010; Lepers et al., 2010, 2016

lactic acid.

Longevity: Tour de France riders live eight years longer, as reported in a major study of athletes and longevity.[15] The age at which 50 percent of the general population died was 73.5 years old, compared to 81.5 years old for Tour de France participants.[16]

Another study observed a 41 percent lower mortality in French cyclists for the main causes of death, including cancer.

Casual cyclists enjoy a 3.7-year longer life expectancy due to the lower stimulus.

(Note that in the following lists, asterisks represent a 1–5 rating system.)

Big muscle groups ****
Low load *****
Huge volume *****
High stimulus. *****
High elasticity *****
MVO2 *****
Longevity *****
Muscle resistance training ***

Hill bounding

Kílian Jornet Burgada and his girlfriend Emelie Forsberg are two of my favorite athletes. Kílian is a modern marvel, able to leap up mountains like a goat and bound down at terrifying speeds. He has the third highest VO2 max ever recorded. Hill bounding or a good stiff hike both task large groups of muscles. Spas like Canyon Ranch in Tucson, Arizona and Rancho La Puerta in Baja California favor hiking, since clients can burn huge amounts of calories and exercise for hours, even with little base training.

Hill bounding is a specialized technique that mimics cross-country skiing. It is an incredibly dynamic sport that builds elasticity,

---

15 https://www.ncbi.nlm.nih.gov/pmc/articles/PMC4534511/
16 https://www.ncbi.nlm.nih.gov/pubmed/21618162

power, and endurance. You drive off the back leg into the air, straightening that leg, pushing your hip forward and lifting your knee high while in the air, and then you land on the ball of your foot. Triathletes and marathoners use this for training, as it is an ideal way to undertake the intensity training needed to boost your MVO2. Here's a video that shows the technique:

https://lydiardfoundation.org/hill-training-the-lydiard-way/

Future US Ski Team stars at Burke Mountain Academy in Vermont focus on hiking in off-season training because of the strength and agility it builds without the injuries of running. (Yuichiro Miura scaled Everest at age 80, his third time since age 70!!!)

Big muscle groups ****
Low load ***
Huge volume ****
High stimulus *****
High elasticity ***
MVO2 *****
Longevity *****
Muscle resistance training ****

Nordic Skiing

Called the Queen of Aerobic Sports, Nordic — or cross-country — skiing requires huge amounts of oxygen because it employs every major and many minor muscle groups through the body. Since the sport involves gliding, there is very little stress on muscles, tendons, or ligaments. The volume of training that skiers undergo is enormous. The key is that much of this is at low intensity, so there is even less stress. The training is varied and highly enjoyable, with some of the best scenery on earth from the towering forests of Royal Gorge Cross Country Ski Resort — the largest cross-country ski area in North America, just over the Donner Pass in California — to the

Alpine peaks surrounding Zermatt, Switzerland. In the off season, you can hill climb, hill bound, or roller ski to deliver high training loads. Nordic skiers have always been at the very top of the VO2 max pyramid and live as long as or longer than many athletes. I love this sport and compete in fourteen races each winter, including the Nordic Masters World Championships and Masters Winter World Games. If you don't live in the snow belt, consider roller skiing and hill bounding. Stand-up paddling is the summer equivalent of Nordic skiing.

Big muscle groups *****
Low load *****
Huge volume *****
High stimulus *****
High spring ***
MVO2 *****
Longevity *****
Muscle resistance training. *****

Rowing

Rowing is called the "King of Aerobic Sports" for its astounding oxygen demands. Rowers also have great longevity, as reported in scientific studies. Rowing uses all major muscle groups, starting with calves, quads, and glutes, and finishing with abdomen, back, and arms. Rowers have the very largest VO2 max of all, as measured by pure volume of oxygen moved in liters per minute.

VO2 max is expressed as milliliters per kilogram (ml/kg), which means the amount of oxygen transported by kilogram of body weight, whereas liters/minute (L/min) determines the raw size of the engine. Steven Rounds Sr., who took up rowing upon retirement at age 66, has won the 2K sprint world title twenty times, and was just seven seconds shy of setting the 2K sprint record for his age group with a time of 8:10.5 at 86 years old — a time many aspiring high school athletes would be proud of. And female rowers live five–seven years longer than the average individual.[17]

---

17 https://www.ncbi.nlm.nih.gov/pubmed/?term=elite+rowing+and+longevity

Big muscle groups *****
Low load *****
Huge volume *****
High stimulus *****
High spring ****
MVO2: *****
Longevity *****
Muscle resistance training *****

Skimo

Ski mountaineering racing, or skimo, is the most fun new sport I've tried, and I've become a huge fan. Skimo allows you to ascend mountains on extremely lightweight racing skis with ribbon-thin climbing skins. At the top of the mountain, you strip off the skins, stash them in your pocket or knapsack, and then descend. You roam far and wide in an alpine environment, one of the greatest joys in sport. The gear section will lay out the best skis for ascending and still getting a great descent.

Big muscle groups *****
Low load *****
Huge volume *****
High stimulus *****
High spring ***
MVO2 *****
Longevity *****
Muscle resistance training ****

Running

Three of the all-time high VO2 max scores were registered by runners: Kílian Jornet Burgada, Jim Ryun, and Joan Benoit Samuelson. Running increases life expectancy — a nearly 50 percent increase with just fifty minutes a day. The trouble with running is that many of us just can't keep up the pace or volume needed over the long term and may ultimately surrender a substantial amount of muscle mass. Sure, those ultra-distance runners built for the event run amazing races late into life. They have incredibly light frames, with less than two pounds per inch of body weight. However, heavier runners get slower and slower with time, lose bounce from their stride, and increase the likelihood of injury.

Have a look at the chart at the below.

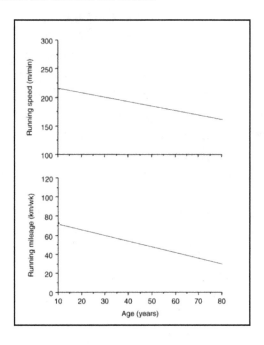

You will see that both running mileage and intensity decrease every decade. This lack of stimulus accounts for the loss of training effect. Simply put, many older runners cannot put in the intensity and mileage as they age because their frames lose the youthful springiness of connective tissue in tendons and ligaments. Their cartilage wears thin in their joints, and they become limited by pain. All of these disadvantages vanish with a change in sport that circumvents this loss of elasticity and bounce. The right sport and gear allow you to apply maximum stimulus and put in all the miles you want. Or, with cross training, you can have several terrific days of intense running and four-five days of recovery in cycling, swimming, or the gym as examples.

Competitive running has a high incidence of hip and knee arthritis, with the risk increasing after fifteen years of running. By the end of my marathon and Ironman career, I had destroyed both hips and had to have them replaced.[18] Curiously, some of those who succeed in running for their whole lives don't develop the arthritis you would expect, given their light frames and superior biomechanics. So, if you continue to be successful at running, keep it up. However, if you can't keep up the intensity of your training, have constant injuries, or overuse syndrome, consider cross training or changing to another sport! When my hips gave out, I changed to cycling, Nordic skiing, and SUP. As a runner you have incredible heart power, which is increasingly trapped by age. Consider harnessing it to sports where you have far better mechanical leverage. The good news? Runners have a 25 percent-40 percent reduced risk of premature mortality and live approximately three years longer than non-runners.[19]

Big muscle groups ***
Low load (0)
Huge volume **
High stimulus ***
High spring (0)
MVO2 ****
Longevity ****
Muscle resistance training *

Walking

Walking ninety minutes a day can result in quite a good benefit — a 35 percent decrease in all-cause mortality. Walking is less efficient than running, attaining the same level of mortality reduction in 105 minutes a day as runners do in twenty-five minutes. Still, if you have

---

18 https://www.ncbi.nlm.nih.gov/pubmed/28504066
19 https://www.ncbi.nlm.nih.gov/pubmed/28365296

the perseverance, walking can be a great activity. Whenever I travel, I get three-five miles a day of walking in addition to my workout. At home I walk my 7-year-old, Alysdair, to the bus every morning. Combine walking with hill bounding for your interval work for an easily available and highly effective combination.

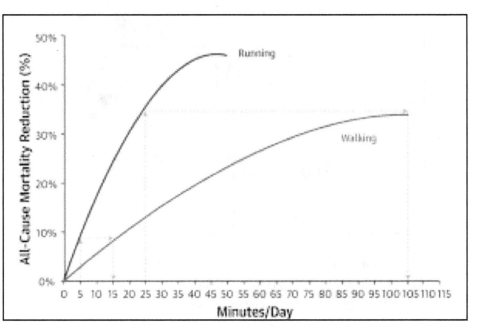

Big muscle groups **
Low load ***
Huge volume **
High stimulus **
High spring (0)
MVO2 ***
Longevity ***
Muscle resistance training *

The Gym

OK. At this point you may be saying, "Hey, I have a life, I can't do these sports. Do I have any hope?" You bet you do! Have a look at this graph showing the increase in life expectancy by just exceeding the modest government fitness guidelines.

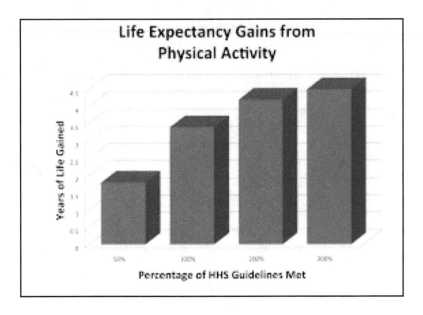

Normal-weight people who exercised for 150 minutes or more weekly lived about 4.7 years longer than normal-weight people who did not do regular moderate exercise, reported by the Harvard School of Public Health. The researchers used data gathered during six previous studies, including a total of nearly 640,000 men and women ages 40 and over. As little as seventy-five minutes of brisk walking a week can increase life expectancy, even for those who are overweight.

"We must not underestimate how important physical activity is for health — even modest amounts can add years to our life," said I-Min Lee MD, ScD of the Harvard School of Public Health.[20]

Leisure-time physical activity is associated with longer life expectancy, even at relatively low levels of activity and regardless of body weight, according to a study by a team of researchers led by the National Cancer Institute. The study, which determined that people who engaged in leisure-time physical activity had life expectancy

---

20 https://www.nurse.com/blog/2012/11/07/even-moderate-physical-activity-boosts-life-expectancy/

gains of as much as 4.5 years.[21] And it's (almost) never too late! Even at the age of 73, regular physical activity can increase life expectancy.[22] I'm still a huge believer, though, of getting outside. As we'll see, those who stuck to the gym had the lowest overall increase in life expectancy.

Your local gym will have equipment that can give you a low-load, high-stimulus workout. Here is some equipment I use:

Treadmill: Set this at 10–15 percent and just do a brisk walk — it doesn't feel hard but burns a ton of calories and gets you fit.

Arc Trainer: This is a high and long step elliptical that engages the biggest muscle groups in lower body.

Concept2 Rowing Ergometer: This device features a fantastic, real rowing-like feel, with a great high load and lowest impact.

Concept2 Wall-mounted Ergometer: This uses the same technology as the rowing ergs, and it is a fantastic device that mimics the double-poling motion of Nordic skiing and SUP.

Ball and Racket Sports

A recent study[23] of Danes revealed that tennis players had a remarkable 9.7 years of additional life. So, why tennis? First, there is a high stimulus with sudden spurts of effort. Second, the authors focused on the social aspects of sport, saying that connecting with other people was an important dimension. We saw that a soccer player had one of the very highest VO2 max scores, and in this study, it added 4.7 years of life. I'm a huge advocate of this social piece of sport. My best social relationships are with my teammates and competitors in sport. Here was the study's final tally, as reported in the Proceedings of the Mayo Clinic:

Tennis: 9.7 years

Badminton: 6.2 years

---

21 http://journals.plos.org/plosmedicine/article?id=10.1371/journal.pmed.1001335

22 https://www.washingtonpost.com/national/health-science/30-minutes-of-exercise-can-increase-lon-gevity-even-if-youre-60-or-70/2015/05/18/f80967ee-fb02-11e4-a13c-193b1241d51a_story.html?utm_term=.33557b0efe8e

23 https://www.mayoclinicproceedings.org/article/S0025-6196(18)30538-X/fulltext

Soccer: 4.7 years
Cycling: 3.7 years
Swimming 3.4 years
Jogging: 3.2 years
Calisthenics: 3.1 years
Health club activities: 3.1 years

In the same study, cyclists gained 3.7 years and joggers just 3.2, though the intensity of these cyclists and runners was thought to be fairly modest. If you observe the speed of the average cyclist in Copenhagen, this could best be described as glacial, since their clunky old bikes don't allow for much speed or intensity. Remember that the Tour de France competitor with a vastly superior volume and intensity of exercise added eight years of life expectancy, demonstrating how vital the right stimulus is. A mix of ball sports with the other aerobic sports is a great plan to keep you engaged and interested in staying fit.

YOUTH IMPROVEMENT TECHNOLOGY

As we've seen, as we age most of us just cannot put on the volume or intensity of training to stay young. That's where great gear comes in. Equipment engineered with the proper ergonometrics, can fit the body like a glove and tremendously leverages the body's ability to work out. My kids know that I am the biggest gearhead of all, because I believe that the gear will take me to the podium! But seriously, great gear helps you get better. Use the gear that world champions use, and it will help teach you to be far better than you imagined. In a nutshell, great gear helps you leverage all your strengths, making you tremendously efficient mechanically and diminishing your weaknesses, so you get just amazing workouts! If I run, I do feel like an old man. I'm slow and can't go more than few miles. But put me on a bike, and I feel like a Tour de France rider. I can ride hundreds of miles and keep up with kids, who are many decades younger. The appendix has my quiver!

CHAPTER 6

INTENSITY!

FOR A LARGE VO2 MAX

"Here comes Diggins. Here comes Diggins, making the play," the announcer screamed hysterically. "Jessie Diggins to the line!"[24] US Ski Team member Jessie Diggins had just won the first Olympic gold medal in the history of US Nordic skiing. "It's not just a medal, it's a gold medal for the United States." How did she do it? A big part was a carefully planned and scientifically based training program.

"It took me many years to understand what my coaches were telling me when they explained that I didn't get faster training," Jesse said. "In fact, they said pounding hours and hours of roller skiing into my body actually slowed me down. I'd just get overtrained, injured, sick, and worst of all, slow."[25]

How you train determines how quickly or slowly you age. Train smart and you not only hold back Father Time by decades, you also recreate youth determined by real physiological metrics. The biggest

24 https://www.adweek.com/brand-marketing/comcast-spliced-footage-of-jessie-diggins-historic-gold-medal-win-into-its-epic-same-day-olympics-spot/
25 https://xcskiworld.com

missing element for the aging athlete is training intensity. We train less, and we train dumb as we age, removing any possibility of a powerful stimulus for youth. It's not that we're destined to fade, it's that we don't have the scientifically backed, professionally designed training program of an athlete like Jessie in her twenties as we get into our thirties, forties, fifties, and beyond. Provide yourself with the same level of intensity as a far younger athlete, and you will succeed past your greatest expectations.

But most of us don't have a real program. We plod through each day, doing exactly the same run, ride, or treadmill/stationary bike workout. Then we get over-trained, as Jessie did. We get injured and frustrated. Then we fade or quit. And most fitness programs involve the same dull plodding every day. The worst are super-high intensity too often, leading to an extraordinary injury rate. A variety of well-honed training programs will spur your interest and make workouts a real pleasure — while creating tremendous improvements.

So, let's look at strategic workouts aimed at improving a specific feature of your performance. Two scientific terms worth learning and that are the language of sport are VO2 max and lactic acid threshold. A progressive reduction in maximal O2 consumption and lactic acid threshold are the primary physiological mechanisms associated with declines in endurance performance with advancing age, and so these are the two most important measures to focus a training program on. This may seem simplistic, but this is the conclusion of decades of scientific study and successful coaching. At the outset, let me say that there are thousands of fantastically talented coaches out there as well as terrific magazines like Runner's World, Bicycling, Women's Running, and Men's Journal that will have far more nuanced tactical and strategic programs that produce great results. What you will read here are the fundamentals of how to improve your physiology to restore youth. Once you have mastered these fundamentals, you may seek more sophisticated training.

The oxygen transport system is the most vital part of increasing your capacity to exercise while attaining a far younger fitness age and improving your life expectancy. Training to improve oxygen transport is aimed at increasing the amount of blood your heart pumps with every beat and delivering the maximum amount of oxygen to working muscles through your body. Typically, these are three-to-five-minute, high-intensity intervals, repeated several times. As part of your training program, undertake this once a week, and you'll find significant gains. A test called maximal O2 consumption (VO2 max) measures this value and should become a vital part of any serious athlete's regular vocabulary. We've already looked at athletes with the very highest VO2 max. To review, here's what you're actually accomplishing:

The heart pumps out more blood with every beat.
The lungs exchange more air, forcing a greater volume of air with
    each breath.
The red blood cells transport more oxygen (top athletes have more
    red blood cells.)

Muscle builds more and larger energy-producing units to offload oxygen and produce power. This is highly specific to the actual part of the muscle used in exercise. For instance, you could be in incredible shape for running, but find you have a low oxygen consumption while cycling, because you haven't trained the segment of the muscle fibers specifically involved. Or you could just train, achieving proficiency at many activities but never enjoying the intensity that benefits you most.

Lactic acid threshold (AT or Anaerobic Threshold): This is the threshold of breathlessness where it becomes difficult to talk and continue to exercise at the same pace. What limits your ability to increase the pace of your workouts across the spectrum of aerobic events — from treadmill and arc climber gym machines to running, cycling, hiking, speed-walking, Nordic skiing, SUP, and rowing — is producing too much lactic acid. Lactic acid begins to fill your muscles, and it decreases the amount of power they can produce. Training at or near the threshold for 20–40 minutes will increase your threshold. For instance, let's say you run a 7:20 mile, and that you're pretty winded at this pace. By training at this 7:20 pace once a week, you'll improve your pace, so that you might run a 6:55 mile before you feel the discomfort of more labored breathing.

The greatest training discovery of the last century for endurance athletes was that this threshold could be measured — and more importantly, increased with training. How does the right training help? Simply, your muscles build more energy without making lactic acid and develop a much greater capacity to suck up the lactic acid that is produced. Typically, my workout will be a steady race pace for twenty-five minutes, once a week. Or I'll add a competition over the weekend at my AT. AT is ordinarily 50 percent of VO2 max for the untrained, and as much as 95 percent for the superbly trained. This means you can use almost all of your VO2 max during a race when you have trained to improve AT. In testing Olympic skiers, I found that the Olympic medalist on our team had an AT at nearly 98 percent of his VO2 max. Totally untrained young skiers were closer to the 50 percent mark. You may have hit the limit on VO2 max years ago but can continue to refine AT each year. I accomplish this by undertaking a time trial on Wednesdays or a race on the weekend.

Suggested stimulus workouts, each once a week:

Twenty minutes at a race-pace time trial
Eight times of three-five-minute intervals, with four minutes rest

Long slow distance (LSD) feels so easy that it's like not training at all, but LSD leads to vast improvements. Why? This milder pace gives your body a chance to fully recover, so that your intense workouts feel easy and even fun to do. You'll be itching to go hard! LSD also allows your body to build up small blood vessels that supply your muscle and the key energy-producing factories in muscle called mitochondria. This is what Jessie does every summer — lots and lots of volume training at slower speeds. LSD is what you want to focus on if you are just starting a sport, so you can build up your muscles, tendons, and ligaments to withstand the strain of more intense workouts. If one mistake is not pushing hard enough, the other is not training slow enough! LSD should be 80 percent of your workouts. If you're just beginning, you'll want months of long-intensity training to prepare your body for higher intensity. You can also cross-train. My SUP coach and current world SUP champion, Michael Booth, likes to train on SUP three times a week and cross-train with running, outrigger paddling, and surf skiing. Yet the SUP workouts are super intense!

Intense intervals: These are the icing on the cake. Intense, fifteen-second to one-minute intervals are easy to do, and they're fun because you go so fast. These intervals improve your neuromuscular coordination and allow you to learn how to go fast. (Always be sure you are warmed up before working these intervals, and then continue at a low pace between them to suck up the lactic acid and decrease the strain on the heart — which doesn't like sudden starting and stopping. If you have heart disease or have not been doing intense exercise, I'd clear these with your MD first and have a formal stress test with an echocardiogram (as I have done).

Weaving these workouts together into a well-thought-out plan is the magic behind training for you. In summary, the reason you may not be succeeding is that you're either not training hard enough ... or easy enough! Do what Olympians do and have a workout program that feels GREAT all the time and delivers spectacular results. The big surprise? This will feel a ton easier than what you may be doing now.

ADVANCED INTERVALS

Fresh challenges make training easier and more fun. I get vastly different kinds of workouts every week, so my training remains interesting. You'll find more advanced intervals to keep things fresh and lend you variety and challenge.

Aerobic power: 2-minute rests
10*4 minutes

12*3 minutes

15*2 minutes

2*4 minutes, 3*3 minutes, 4*2 minutes

Anaerobic power: 2-minute rests

10*1 minute

8*75 seconds

15*45 seconds

Neuromuscular power: Allow a good recovery between each so that you are applying full power. Stop when your power or speed starts to decline. A minute or so is a good interval between them.

10*15 seconds

15*30 seconds

10*20 seconds

Lactate Tolerance

15*30 seconds, 15 seconds rest

15*45 seconds, 15 seconds rest

15*20 seconds 10 seconds rest

You can slot these in as alternative interval workouts in your weekly programs, providing more variety. You want three interval workouts a week, maximum.

The five biggest training mistakes

1. No easy training
2. No intervals
3. Overuse and injury
4. Unchanged daily or weekly workouts
5. The wrong activity

GOALS

1—The Novice

If you train very little or not at all, the key to a great program is making it easy and enjoyable. You will make regular and spectacular gains, but the worst thing you can do is push too hard and become over-trained or even injured. This is one of the best things you will ever do for yourself, extending your longevity, increasing your youthfulness, and decreasing the risk of chronic illness.

Start slow: Your body needs the time to make stronger ligaments, tendons, and joints. There's no need for intensity to begin with as you create a solid platform. Many great Olympic training programs begin with building volume at a slow pace to create a solid foundation. Take a day or two completely off each week.
Build fitness into your day: I get lots of extra exercise every day by just walking. In New York City, as one example, I'll walk between appointments, and find I often have logged an extra three to eight miles a day. My favorite expression is, "Work while you're working out if you really can't find the time." Walk on a treadmill at an incline and bring along your iPad or iPhone to catch up on emails or read for work or entertainment. The time will fly by, and you'll pack in much of the volume you need.

Mix it up: The body is extremely sensitive to overuse as you begin a new program or increase volume or intensity. I'll mix up ellipticals, treadmills, using the rowing machine, walking, and hiking to just build volume and take the stress off of sore joints and ligaments. You'll dramatically decrease your chance of injury and of getting stale. Recover! The lesson that some Olympic athletes are still learning is recovery. Taking a day or two off a week allows lots of time for your body to rebuild and incorporate all its gains. Easy days help you build for the future. Remember you are building a platform onto which you want to place your key VO2 max workouts. This platform has to be solid, and it has to be broad. When I trained Olympic ski racers, my most challenging job was holding racers back! You only need two intense days a week.

2—The Master

As a Master, you've achieved much of the dream of lifelong youth. You may be slowing down at the sport you've devoted decades to and be up for a new challenge that will reinvigorate you. Or you may want to take advantage of the new research in exercise physiology and the new gear and tech that will allow you to accelerate your current performance. I met with a group of elite Rhode Island runners in their mid-thirties. Even at that young age range, they could sense they were slowing down, reducing their mileage, and losing race speed. I explained how they still had a spectacular heart-lung package but needed to harness it to a sport that allowed them to use their full potential. Most were eager for a transition to embrace their dreams of victory. Leverage your talents to apply the maximum stimulus to your training each week and select new sports where you may gain even greater advantages. Focus on high stimulus and great recoveries. Consider dynamic training (in the coming chapter) to improve your practice and really crush it!!!

3—The Artisan

Artisanal athletes have made a craft out of their sport. Like a fine workman, the artisan has carefully assembled the finest tools of the sport, enhancing performance, safety, and enjoyment. But the artisan also recognizes that much of the true joy in sport comes from the continual improvement in technique and training. Every day I find great joy in learning something new in my sports. Technical mastery in sport is one of life's great joys. If you're currently a Master in running or a non-technical endurance sport, I'd strongly encourage you to look at mastering a more technical sport. You may flounder at the beginning. I sure did. But each day and week, you'll steadily improve. If you race, you'll find that you slowly become a true professional. You may make many blunders to start, from falling at the beginning of a race to making tactical mistakes or "bonking" as your blood sugar plummets due to a lack of fuel. Sport becomes a great surrogate for life. The triumph you have in sport translates to daily life. You can have a bad day at work but a great day training, giving yourself an added sense of achievement.

TRAINING PROGRAMS

I've always found training programs a mystery. Why did a coach pick a certain distance or pace? I wrote this section to demystify training. Across all endurance sports there are only four important kinds of training, each with a fundamental biological basis and a highly specific physiological goal, tightly linked to athletic success and long-term longevity and fitness.

1—Training Intensity: Stimulus

The Freshness Principle: Muscles respond best to a training stimulus when they are fresh, and your nervous system is rested. My SUP coach, Michael Booth, told me, "I only train hard when I feel great." You can do the same by only training hard on days when you are superbly recovered.

Green: This is slow, comfortable training, designed to harden your tendons, joints, and ligaments so they can handle the load of greater training intensity. You'll also slowly grow capillaries and the small energy factories in your muscle. This training should always feel easy and relaxing. No need to push. In fact, I don't want you to push at all. Hold yourself back. The only mistake you can make is not going slow enough. This leaves you fresh enough for your harder workouts. This is usually called long slow distance, or LSD.

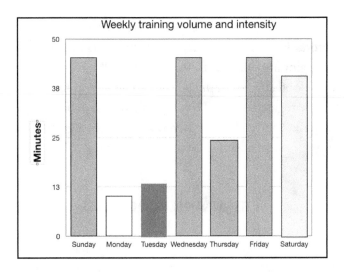

Yellow: This is the pace where you're just starting to get short of breath. This trains your body to handle lactic acid much better, so you can go faster and faster with time. We call this race pace, and it is what you would run a 10k race at. Aim for twenty minutes and build to thirty or forty.

Orange: This is the sweet spot and final goal of all your training, to push your VO2 max upward, with intervals of three-five minutes in duration, just the right amount to maximally tax your heart and lungs. In the training plan, you can see that this follows a very easy day, so that you are ready to crush it! Start by doing five three-minute intervals once a week.

Red: These genius intervals will train your neuromuscular system to go faster and also help improve VO2 max. These thirty-second intervals are also at the heart of HIIT training, which achieves VO2 increases comparable to the longer three-five-minute intervals. Do these intervals once a week. They follow a complete day off, so that you are itching to work out.

This illustration demonstrates how these intervals might be deployed over the course of a week, following the color chart from above. LSD pre-dominates, providing lots of rest and recovery to be able to hit your yellow, orange, and red days with vigor! As you can observe, this chart shows how hard days might be deployed within a sea of green (easy recovery) days to derive maximum benefit.

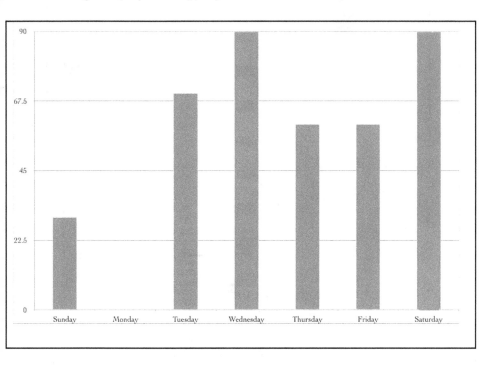

2—Weekly Training Amounts and Intensity

Now let's see how this translates into a week of training in even greater detail. The height of the columns represents the number of minutes of exercise. The red color corresponds to the length of the interval. You can see there are only three days a week of intense training for a high-end Master athlete.

For routine fitness, there are only two, the three-minute and the thirty-second intervals. The length of the red bar shows the time of the interval. For instance, on Tuesdays nine small bars signify thirty-second intervals. Wednesdays have longer red bars, signifying three-five-minute intervals. Saturdays has one long red interval signifying a

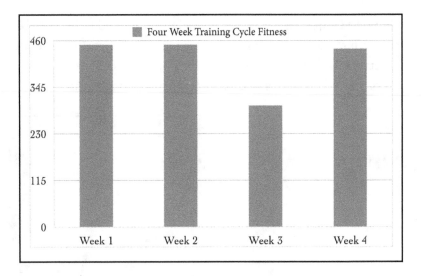

twenty-five-minute anaerobic threshold interval. The pure blue bars on Sunday, Thursday, and Friday signify easy workouts.

The following chart breaks the workouts into finer detail, showing the length of intervals relative to the total workout time.

3—Monthly Training Amounts

Just as intensity and training volume vary within a week, you will want to vary your total training volume on a week-to-week basis over several months. This allows you to build great strength and endurance while building in time to recover. These are called macrocycles. For most athletes, a two-week on one-week lower intensity and volume cycle makes sense, according to long-time ironman coach John Spinney. More elite athletes could opt for three weeks on and one week of lower intensity.

4—Sample Week

Sunday: Long, slow distance. Enjoy the day. No need to push. Really do go slow to recover. Focus on each part of your movement to improve. For instance, with paddling, focus first on sliding your paddle into the water without a splash for ten minutes. Then take ten minutes to focus on the pull.

	% Maximum HR	How you feel
Very light	<57	
		Very light
Light	57-63	
		Fairly light
Moderate	64-76	
		Somewhat hard
Vigorous	77-95	
		Very hard
Near Maximal	>96	
		>very hard

Monday: Rest. This is the hardest thing for any athlete to do. Enjoy the day off. You're letting your body rebuild. If you still want to work out, take on another activity, like an elliptical trainer or treadmill, to burn calories—but for no more than thirty minutes and at a very low intensity.

Tuesday: This is the most fun day of the week, with short intervals that vastly improve your technique, power, strength, resilience, and timing. Have an easy workout between these intervals. You'll finish refreshed and strong. (Example: thirty seconds as hard as you can go, two minutes off, then repeat. A total of six thirty-second intervals are also a highly effective way of increasing your VO2 max. I do 15*1 minute and 15*30 second intervals for world championship SUP training.)

Wednesday: Today is built around building more heart and lung power, with longer intervals designed to push your heart and lungs to deliver the most oxygen of all. Ordinarily, you might find workouts like this hard. However, after a several days of rest and easy recovery, these will feel easy. This is the most important day in your week, since this most effectively pushes up VO2 max. Try to do four intervals of three minutes each at maximum intensity. Be careful to ease into these, or you'll max out early and not get the full value. This is the best day to use the Humon Hex or Moxy SmO2 device if you have one. Do two minutes in the green and the last in the orange or red. I do 14*4 minutes one week and 14*5 minutes the following week.

Thursday: Focus on technique during these long, slow recovery distance days. I take Olympic gold-medal canoeist Larry Cain's advice when paddling and focus on each aspect of the stroke for ten minutes.

Friday: Focus on long, slow distance. If you have a race or fun competition on Saturday, either take the day off or do an alternative activity, such as cycling.

Saturday: This is your anaerobic threshold day. Do twenty minutes at race pace. Masters should aim for thirty-forty minutes. (This is at the point where you're just starting to get breathless.) Or substitute a competition. With a Humon Hex, just touch orange and back off ever so slightly to stay in the green.

Duration

You'll want to slowly work up to large volumes, with much less emphasis on intensity, until you are comfortable with the volume you are going to stick with. This is how we will build your long, slow distance days.

Month 1: Long 30-45 minutes
Month 2: Long 1 hour
Month 4: Long 1 hour 15 minutes
Month 6: Long 1 hour 30 minutes

OK!!! So this may sound complex; however, training technology has leveled the playing field to make world-class training equally accessible to all athletes, from Novice to Master. You'll see that this is as simple as just slotting your two or three high-intensity days into the days when you are highly recovered and have the full resources to totally crush your workout.

MEASURES OF INTENSITY

The last piece of a precise training prescription determines exactly how hard to train on your hard days. Since the higher-intensity workout proves so critically important to developing a large VO2 max, let's look at the key methods for you to choose from in determining pace.

These are the time-tested principles: perceived exertion, pace in running, power in cycling, time in rowing pieces, anaerobic threshold determination, and heart rate. There is also the new emerging technology of muscle oxygen consumption, which we'll look at last and which may prove the most effective.

NOVICE

1. Perceived Exertion: One of the oldest measures of intensity, this relies on how hard you feel you are working out. The biggest danger here is that during an interval you may quickly reach an all-out ten in the first few seconds because you have gone too hard, and then spend the rest of the interval recovering. However, with pacing, you'll get a sense of how hard you are working out. This is the least precise method.

2. Heart Rate Zones: Heart rate has become the most popular means of determining workout pace for many athletes. The key in establishing your heart rate train zones is beginning with the

Level	Name Purpose	Effort	Time
1	LSD	3	1 hour
2	Lactate Threshold	5	30 minutes
3	VO2Max	6	5 minutes
4	Anaerobic Capacity	7	30 second

maximum predicted heart rate for your age. You'll determine an average value, since some very fit athletes may maintain a higher maximum heart rate later into life. The basic formula for a generation has simply been 220 minus your age. So, if you are fifty, 220 minus 50 yields a maximum heart rate of 170. There are then several methods of determining where your high, medium, and low training ranges are. The Karvonen[26] method is more sophisticated, since this method incorporates both your maximum heart rate and your resting heart rate.

Basic versus Karvonen: The Karvonen yields much higher and more realistic training zones. Take the hard-anaerobic zone as an example. The Karvonen yields 127-137—right about where I train—whereas the basic method yields 119-135. The moderate training zone, where you'll spend most of your time, is 116-127 with Karvonen but just 104-119 with the standard method. By using resting heart rate, Karvonen accounts for your actual physiology to a greater degree than the basic method. Whichever method you use, you'll establish your own training zones more accurately through training.

---

26 https://www.calculatorsoup.com/calculators/health/target-heart-rate-zone-calculator.php

Target Zone	% Intensity	THR in bpm Karvonnen MHR RHR	Basic
Maximum VO2 Max Zone	90% - 100%	137 - 147	134 - 149
Hard Anaerobic Zone	80% - 90%	127 - 137	119 - 134
Moderate Aerobic Zone	70% - 80%	116 - 127	104 - 119
Light Fat Burn Zone	60% - 70%	106 - 116	89 - 104

Where heart rate works:

I like heart rate for steady state work. That is, if I'm competing in a ten-mile SUP competition, I'll peg my heart rate at 147 and keep it there. If I start to slack off, I can see that on my Garmin and increase my pace. If the workload becomes higher, such as when racing into stiff wind and big waves, my heart rate may fall, since the load is more muscular than cardiovascular, so I'll shorten my stroke to lighten the muscular load and put the load back onto my cardiovascular system. Another example is cycling into a stiff wind in a high gear — lower the gearing to keep your heart rate up. I like heart rate best as a way of assessing if I am applying my full cardiovascular power to an activity.

Where heart rate fails:

Intervals: Heart rate responds too slowly to be of value in shorter intervals. For instance, in a one-minute interval, heart rate keeps climbing even after the interval is completed. Even though you may exert maximum intensity, your heart rate may fail to climb, since the aerobic load is so low. You may use heart rate to gauge recovery, allowing it to fall below 100 before beginning your next interval.

Day to day variation: I'll find heart rate is quite different from one day to the next at exactly the same speed or intensity. Part of this is not enjoying a full recovery, so that the heart is not ready to respond. One theory is that the beta receptors on the heart, which respond to adrenalin and sympathetic tone, are diminished after a hard workout and take a day or so to reconstitute. I find that with a scientifically designed program, heart rates can be pretty accurate if you're going all out after a full recovery. Then, if you are recovered and your muscles are relaxed and fueled, your heart rate should respond maximally. Still, you have to work with a very consistent pace for heart rate to have meaning.

ADVANCED

3. Anaerobic threshold: This is the most critical pace to determine an accurate measure, so you can design your training program around it. Commonly, this would be the heart rate where you can hold a steady pace for twenty minutes or more while right on the verge of breathlessness—after a great recovery. We used to determine this in my lab using a breath-by-breath gas exchange system. This signaled when the body began to expel massive amounts of carbon dioxide because of the quickly rising amounts of lactic acid in the bloodstream. We also directly measured lactic acid by taking blood samples. The East Germans pioneered direct anaerobic threshold measurements in training and won multiple gold medals in rowing by knowing precisely how much lactic acid was being produced and at which points during a 2,000-meter race, then using the information tactically to win.

Determining threshold:[27] Cycling coach Joe Friel has a great quick guide to setting up zones.

1. Race as hard as you can for an entire thirty-minute period in your chosen endurance sport.
2. Click the lap button on your heart rate monitor at ten minutes.

---

27 https://www.trainingpeaks.com/blog/joe-friel-s-quick-guide-to-setting-zones/

When you are finished, take the average heart rate for the last twenty minutes. This is your threshold heart rate. How do you know you are going fast enough? Fast enough that you can't say but a few words however you still experience deep, steady and even breathing.

3. Now you or your coach can divide your training into specific physiologic zones, which would look like the ones in the accompanying graphic. Threshold refers to anaerobic threshold. You'll want to determine a heart rate zone associated with each of these. This test determines a pace right between sub-threshold and super-threshold. Training categories then are constructed as you'll see in this chart, showcased above and below the threshold pace you have determined.

Zone	Name
1	Recovery
2	Aerobic
3	Tempo
4	Subthreshold
5A	Super threshold
5B	Aerobic Capacity
5C	Anaerobic Capacity

4. Strain: Fitness training program WHOOP employs artificial intelligence to demonstrate how much strain your body can take each morning. WHOOP has taken at least three weeks to learn about you and generate useful strain estimates. While strain doesn't designate an actual intensity, you can review your workout afterward and see how close you came to the strain that WHOOP advised. For instance, I'll see an "18 strain" recommendation, then go all out in a two-hour SUP race at near maximum heart rate. After the race, WHOOP calculates the actual strain to see if the projected strain meets your actual strain. You'll learn over time to hit that mark pretty accurately.

I reviewed this concept with Olympic gold medalist Larry Cain. Larry told me it just doesn't make sense to strain the body when it can't take the strain, so having an actual recommendation based on your recovery becomes a big step forward. Peak strain may be achieved best in the late afternoon when all your body hormones are in perfect alignment after a great recovery day.

5. Pace: Rowing, running, swimming, and other sports have very precise metrics to determine an exact pace for an athlete's training. Runners know their pace within seconds per mile and will be given workouts based on highly specific minute-per-mile paces, say 6:20 miles for four miles after a warmup. Rowers will also be given specific times to meet for "pieces" ranging from 500–2,000 meters and beyond, both on the water and in the ergometer. A beginner might be lucky to break eight minutes for 2,000 meters on the water, an erg, or rowing machine. The world champion can hit 5:35!!!

6. Power: Cyclists are incredibly lucky to have power meters built into the hubs or crank arms of bikes; they are the best fitness devices you can add to your bike. Workouts are then set up and measured in watts. For instance, I'll run my three-minute intervals at 300 watts. I'll do my thirty-second intervals at 600 watts. Over time, I can see how the power improves. Whether you have a headwind or pedaling uphill, the power meter still accurately reflects your power output.

7. GPS Speed: SUP, kayak, Nordic, ski mountaineering racing, and canoe athletes also have precise pace based on GPS measurement systems that allow them to mark out specific workouts. Garmin Forerunner watches have paces for running, rowing, and even SUP, so you can watch your pace in real time. Variable terrain, wind, and current make speed a less-consistent measurement.

ELITE

8. SmO2 (You may skip this section if you do not have an SmO2 device)

The heart of this book is growing the largest aerobic power at the highest sustainable intensity. We've looked at all the standard metrics for intensity: heart rate, pace, power meters, etc. However, none of these show you the most important metrics of all: real-time oxygen consumption or anaerobic threshold. Humon Hex and Moxy have invented ingenious wearable devices that measure both real-time muscle oxygen saturation and anaerobic threshold. I've used both in my training.

Theory: Near infrared sensors look down into your muscle to see how much oxygen is present. (Technically, these sensors look for hemoglobin that is carrying oxygen.) As you observe increased exercise intensity, you can see the amount of oxygen your muscle is consuming. During an interval, muscle oxygen drops to the point that there is little oxygen left, demonstrating how much oxygen your muscle consumes in real time.

Strategic value: SmO2 becomes the most important single aspect of your entire effort to develop a large VO2 max, since there is so much room to improve SmO2 at any age. Why? Heart and lung performance, as we have seen, peak in your late teens, if you've trained all your life. Otherwise, heart and lung power peak after two to three years of training. The great news is that this is not the end of your ability to enjoy tremendous gains by building the energy producing machinery inside your muscle cells. SmO2 looks directly into your muscle cells to observe this and assists you in training them optimally. Improving the demand side of VO2 max from the muscle itself is where all the gains are made later in life. Moxy CEO Roger Schmitz told me, "At its heart, SMO2 allows you to see in real time how your physiology is limiting your performance, viewing the balance between oxygen supply and demand in the muscle. You can observe how the athlete responds to training loads and how they fatigue." You'll develop phenomenal insights as you use SmO2 more and more during training and competition.

Relation to exercise physiology: These amazing devices get close to the point they can measure when the muscle goes anaerobic. When your muscle cells can no longer find any oxygen stores inside the muscle cell or in nearby blood vessels, the cell switches to making energy without oxygen. Energy production becomes severely limited over a short time interval because the muscle produces a toxic acid called lactate, which will quickly builds in your muscle cells. The actual acidity starts to shut down all of the energy-producing machinery in the cell, and you will slow to an abrupt halt or dramatically decrease your intensity as you become markedly short of breath and your muscles begin to burn.

How this helps: As you monitor muscle oxygen consumption while you train, you'll learn to apply exactly the right stimulus for your muscle cells to build massive amounts of energy production. This improves your pace in training and racing and your VO2 max. You'll learn when you are at precisely the limit of exertion. By completely emptying your cells of oxygen, you'll be able to build stunning anaerobic power.

Humon Hex: This device has a much tighter scale, say 68–76. The Humon Hex has an ingenious software program that shows when you start to run out of oxygen (orange), and when you have solidly hit your anaerobic threshold (red). Tests have put these devices up against actual lactate measurements. While not extremely precise, they are uncanny in the practical world of training and racing, since you'll rapidly experience shortness of breath and fatigue when you hit red.

Moxy: This device has a larger range to follow than Humon Hex. For instance, I'll start a workout at 60 and be able to drive my oxygen consumption down to 26 when my muscle is bereft of any oxygen stores.

Scale:
Low: 26
High: 76

How to Use SmO2

Humon Hex: This comes with a Velcro strap that wraps around your quads. Be sure to download the Humon drivers from the Garmin website and install them on you Garmin watch. Then, pick either the Humon interval or endurance field for the activity you're undertaking (e.g., SUP, cycling). Next, turn the device on once with a hard press of the button on top of the device, then two short presses. Be sure you see a reading on your watch. The light should turn blue, then green, and you should see a reading on your Garmin watch. I put my Garmin on my SUP board, Nordic ski, or bicycle handlebar so I can watch SmO2 in real time. Extremely cool!!!

> **Color scheme:**
> Green: normal oxygen consumption
> Orange: lessened oxygen consumption
> Red: little oxygen left, at anaerobic threshold and pushing beyond
> Turquoise: recovery

Moxy: These are tricky to put on your body. They come with a white tape that does stick well to the skin, but you have to be very careful it doesn't get tangled up as you apply it. It takes a few tries to get right. Moxy also offers Lycra shorts to hold the device on. I've only used it on my quads, but in theory you could affix the Moxy to any muscle. You'll want to turn the device on and be sure it's working with your Garmin or wearable before attaching it to your body. You'll see an oxygen reading come up immediately when it's working properly. Turn the device over and look at the bottom for a red blinking light.

Here are some specific applications of SmO2:

1. How to warm up: Warmup has less to do with the actual temperature of the muscle and more with blood flow, as you redirect blood flow to exercising muscles and dilate the arteries to allow more blood flow. With SmO2, you can watch the oxygen saturation rise during your warmup. When it reaches maximum, you are ready for your workout. I'll find I need as much as a half hour to really get warmed up. Proper warmup lends you much higher intensities during your workout and lessens your risk of injury. You do not want to go anaerobic early in a workout. However, you do want to go as hard as you can without going anaerobic if you want to warm up quickly before an event or competition.

Steepness: You'll develop tremendous insights as you observe both fast descents in muscle oxygen levels during intervals and slower descents for AT and aerobic workouts. You'll find what you can tolerate and withstand in terms of demanding interval and race paces. You may replay these on your iPhone, observing the steepness or shallowness of the descent curve.

2. Improve VO2 max: We've seen that the three-five-minute interval gives the muscle the greatest stimulus to improve VO2 max. However, applying this training stimulus evenly for maximum benefit has been very tricky. With SmO2, I've observed that I can drive my muscle oxygen consumption down dramatically in the first fifteen seconds, then observe the muscle recover over the next several minutes rather than remaining low. In other words, I didn't really do a three-minute interval, I did a fifteen-second interval and recovered for two minutes and forty-five seconds. With SmO2 I start the interval more judiciously, driving SmO2 down slowly for the first two minutes, then hit the red line in the last minute and try to hold till the end of the interval. This provides the maximum stimulus to the enzyme system in your muscles to build the maximum aerobic power. With the Humon Hex, as soon as you see orange, back off just slightly so you're in the green or verging on orange, but not red. With Moxy you'll want to learn what your range is. For instance, I'll drive mine from fifty down to thirty-two for two minutes, then drive down to twenty-six for the last minute.

3. Build anaerobic threshold: We've seen that anaerobic threshold is the most important training concept of the last half century. Raising anaerobic threshold allows you to use a higher and higher percentage of your VO2 max and compete or train at a faster and faster pace. With SmO2 you can observe the precise point pace that you can hold for twenty to thirty minutes and attempt to hold exactly that pace. When you begin using SmO2, you'll develop many insights. For instance, you'll see large variations in SmO2 as you push too hard. Or you may find that you haven't been pushing hard enough to reach threshold. We ran a race with $300,000 worth of gear to test AT with US Ski Team athletes. To be able to get the same values in training with extremely lightweight variables becomes a staggering advance for those of us who pioneered the use of AT in training. Select a value to hold on the Moxy. Hold orange on the Humon Hex or into the green below orange.

4. Anaerobic Power: To make shorter (fifteen-second to one-minute) intervals really count, drive your SmO2 as low as you can. Combined with power and pace outputs, you'll ensure that you're getting as much as you can out of an interval. Heart rate won't be able to respond nearly fast enough to show how hard you are going.

5. HIIT: High intensity interval training has gained enormous popularity for the time constrained. Here's how I do them. Go the fastest pace or highest power setting you can and try to drive SmO2 into the red, so there is little oxygen left and you are training your body to learn how to produce anaerobic power. The thirty-second interval is the heart of HIIT training, which shows similar increases in VO2 max to longer intervals. For HIIT, you'd typically have thirty seconds on, twenty seconds off, for a total of five minutes after a good warmup. This is a grueling but highly efficient workout and is becoming increasingly popular.[28] You can observe recovery in the twenty-second-off period, then drive your SmO2 down again.[29] HIIT has many variations, and there are many great gyms that teach the various methods.

---

28 https://en.wikipedia.org/wiki/High-intensity_interval_training
29 https://en.wikipedia.org/wiki/High-intensity_interval_training

6. Recovery: This is easy to gauge with SmO2, since you can watch your oxygen levels rise into a recovery range. For instance, I'm 68 percent for a tempo pace, 57 percent for a very hard short interval, and 75 percent for recovery. Once I see 75 percent, I know it's time to hammer again! This occurs a minute or more before my heart rate recovers, so I have a faster interval turnover. On the Humon Hex, you'll see the device turn turquoise to show you are in the recovery range.

7. Muscle Balance: Place the SmO2 sensor on different sides of your body during a workout and look at the difference in SmO2 for a series of intervals. You'll likely find a muscle imbalance, which you may remedy by applying a higher load to the weaker muscle. So, for cyclists or runners, try one quad and then the other to see if there is a difference at precisely the same pace.

8. Systemic balance: A unique phenomenon of SmO2 measurement is that you will find a drop in a muscle group that you are not heavily engaging. For instance, in cycling you may max out your quads and hardly be using your arms at all. However, SmO2 will drop as the more active muscles "steal oxygen" from the arms, says Moxy's Roger Schmitz.

Regarding overall advantages of SmO2, here's what Roger told me: "SmO2 lets you see inside the body in real time. You don't need to be in a lab. Swimmers wear Moxy in the water, Motocross riders on a dirt track; SmO2 really changed things, since you can see inside your muscles while you exercise. SmO2 allows you to infer a huge amount of information, including anaerobic and ventilatory thresholds."

SmO2 Practical Examples

Cycling 1: One-minute intervals: My coach assigned me ten one-minute bike intervals. At the beginning of each one, I dug in and spun the power up to 600 watts. My heart rate began at 80 and reached 94. But within fifteen seconds, the Humon turned a bright red. I was in severe oxygen debt. This taught me several lessons. First, high power at the beginning of the interval meant petering out in the remaining forty-five seconds. Better to build into the interval with a shallower descent in SmO2. This reading also demonstrated that I had done my very, very best!!!

Cycling 2: Fifteen-minute intervals: During a ninety-minute ride, my coach had me perform all-out fifteen-minute intervals. Yet what is "all-out"? How can you be certain you don't spike at the beginning and then drift off? When the ride began, my SmO2 was 59, a sure sign that a warmup would help a lot. After twenty-five minutes, SmO2 reached the mid-seventies. Then I cranked up the power to 300 and watched the SmO2 drop to 72, where it steadied out. On the steeper hills, SmO2 dropped to 68, and the screen went from green to a bright red, meaning I crossed the anaerobic threshold. Continuing at that pace would create tremendous fatigue, so I backed off to the border between orange and green on the Humon Hex. This created the greatest demand for oxygen and the greatest stimulus to make more powerful chemicals as a result of the training. On downhills, when it was impossible to keep the power up, the SmO2 drifted up into the recovery range, 76, a turquoise color. This recovery means there's no training stimulus. In the end, this workout became much more productive because of the even pacing and maximum stimulus. Without the SmO2, pacing would prove to be far more challenging. Heart rate proved so slow to respond to the small drops or rises in power that it proved of no value. SmO2 allows you to enjoy the very highest benefits possible from a workout.

Cross-country skiing: Hills: The big hill on the C loop of the Masters World Championship course in Norway was like climbing a wall on skis. I wore my Humon Hex device and observed the colors: green, orange, and red. As I slammed into the bottom of the hill at full effort, the screen went from green to orange to red. I became acutely short of breath. Without the Humon, I would have pushed up the hill at that pace, figuring I was putting in a full effort and going as fast as possible. But knowing that the Humon showed me little oxygen left in my muscle, I knew the effort was futile and backed off to an orange reading, maintaining that pace up the hill, allowing me to then pass half a dozen people. SmO2 fundamentally changes how you approach hills in any sport. You'll see that too much early effort can destroy your performance, flooding your muscles with lactic acid. By backing off slightly to just under AT, you can find a terrific pace that you can maintain up the hill. As you approach the crest, push yourself back into the red and use the downhill to actively recover.

SUP: Four-minute intervals: Each week on Wednesday I spar with three-time Olympian Tommy Buday. We choose a four-minute interval. Before SmO2, I would dig in hard and even pull slightly ahead in the opening minute, then fall progressively further behind as my shoulders tightened with pain and fatigue. With SmO2, I'd get a good start but keep myself aerobic for the first three minutes. On the Humon Hex, that meant just touching orange and backing off. With Moxy, I'd drop SmO2 to 32 percent, but no lower, then in the last-minute drop into the red on the Humon or 25 percent on the Moxy. I could increase my pace as I went deeply anaerobic to get the very most out of the interval. By keeping yourself just out of the red zone for the first several minutes of a longer interval, you're triggering the very highest production of aerobic power generation in your muscle.

Q&A:

What if you don't see any drop at all? If you're new to intensive training, you may not be able to generate much of a drop. However, with time this will improve, with more and more intervals to stress your muscles.

CHAPTER 7

DYNAMIC TRAINING

TRAIN EASILY LIKE A PRO FOR GREAT RESULTS

From the 19-year-old Olympic wanna-be to the average middle-aged athlete, many of us just pound away day after day and week after week at almost the same pace. We're sore, overtrained, sleeping poorly, eating badly, and losing fitness. A great local friend in his early sixties bikes, runs, hikes and plays tennis but complains of feeling sore and old every day. I told him that the solution is dynamic training, which properly balances strenuous and easy days so he can recover and ease the soreness. Dynamic training may sound like a daunting solution, but it feels sooooo much easier and is incredibly effective. By having really hard days, really easy days, and even rest days, I upped my fitness dramatically while easing my chronic overtraining and flipping the youth switch. All good training programs vary between hard and easy days. However, I have found that there is no way to know which training day should be hard or easy. You may blunder into missing an amazing high recovery day when you could completely crush a great workout, or you may have very low recovery days where you try to push yourself without benefit and with the risk of injury, illness, or overtraining. With Heart Rate Variability (HRV) you can visualize the amazing high recovery days when you can push yourself to the limit. Should you not recover well, you may benefit from several easy days. As we've seen, World SUP champion Michael Booth says, "I only train when I feel good!" And Michael wins more consistently than anyone!

Dynamic training is vastly simpler, easier, and more pleasurable than any previous training program and a big improvement to the training programs we have just looked at, if you are willing to measure HRV.

Before diving into dynamic training, let's take a more in-depth look at HRV, since this measurement underlines dynamic training, rest, restoration, and the reconstruction of youth by restoring the proper balance of high and low HRVs.

HRV

Cooked!!! In 2019 I competed in the master's world championships for cross-country skiing in Norway, racing 10 km, 15 km, and 30 km events against the best in the world from Russia, Norway, Sweden, Switzerland, and the US, then polished off the trip with a winter ski mountaineering ascent of the highest local mountain with the chief local guide. Barely able to walk and unable to bend my knees due to excruciating pain, I was completely trashed after the trip home. My fiancé said, "You look like an old man. You're hunched over, you need help getting out of a chair, no one would know you're an athlete." She was right! I'd massively overdone it and was overtrained, or as coaches like to say, "cooked." Through my whole life, I'd never been able to figure out the right balance of training and rest, and I was now paying a heavy price. I resolved to search for a coach who could help master recovery, and I found that coach in John Spinney, a high-performance coach across several brands at QT2 Systems LLC, where he has coached for ten years. A major component of John's coaching is his focus on helping his athletes to create and maintain the "daily performance environment." John has competed in hundreds of bike races and running races plus over 200 triathlons since the age of 14, including thirteen ironmans, and twice competed at the Ironman World Championship in Hawaii.

I'd met him at a ski mountaineering racing camp.

"How can I help?" John queried.

"Better prediction of overtraining," I countered.

"Get a WHOOP," John told me.

After some initial research, I discovered that WHOOP is a system across software, hardware, and analytics that improves human performance.

This fantastically accurate device precisely measures sleep, training, rest, and a critical important new metric, HRV. Combining HRV with sleep, resting heart rate, and daily strain, the WHOOP tells you every morning whether you are fully recovered to crush it (green), not fully rested but still ready for a good workout (yellow), or fried (red) and in need of a day off. Heart rate variability is becoming the most powerful marker of day-to-day youth, health, and fitness. There are several different devices and good phone apps. However, after testing many different systems of measuring HRV, I found only HRV on the WHOOP is reproducible day after day.

WHOOP

Founder and CEO Will Ahmed told me he wanted to take the precision of the finest $20,000 EKG, take measurements 100 times a second, and implant it in a wearable wrist strap. As a Harvard college student and competitive squash player, Ahmed pondered a vexing problem. Day after day, athletes were running themselves down, with no guidelines to balance stress and recovery. Some were sidelined for months. He wanted to measure strain and recovery and present those measurements on a platform that athletes could use to improve their training programs while avoiding the curse of overtraining. Will emphasized that for generations, athletes believed they could feel when they were recovered and when they were overtrained. The data showed a different story. While the body could signal recovery and overtraining, these were not sensations that an athlete could accurately sense. Sophisticated technology would be required to determine these values. As a Harvard Squash Team captain, he had hundreds of friends who were overtrained and without a solution. He developed a method and founded WHOOP as a result. His most famous quote is, "You can ONLY manage what you can measure." So, I could finally manage overtraining and recovery! Will has millions of hours of athlete data and has been remarkably helpful to scores of professional and amateur athletes. As an example, using WHOOP, a top NBA player scored more points per game when he was able to determine he was fully recovered. Will has an amazing Podcast series featuring a wide spectrum of athletes that you'll find both highly inspirational and quite helpful in your own training. I've listened to and enjoyed the entire series.

Sports scientists have long considered the ability to identify overtraining as a holy grail precisely because athletes and coaches cannot pinpoint it on their own. "I realized overtraining was an imbalance between stress and recovery. Day after day you are running your body down," Will said.

I was sold on the concept, and soon a UPS truck arrived with my WHOOP. Ripping the box open with wild anticipation, I found the device encased like a fine piece of jewelry in a round red base below a clear display case. It easily clasped around my wrist, and I found that WHOOP records a highly detailed record of my beat-to-beat heart rate, sleep quality, strain, and other variables. This is uploaded constantly to WHOOP headquarters, where a brilliant team of world-class data and physiology scientists continually analyze the results and upgrade the product.

ARTIFICIAL INTELLIGENCE AT ITS BEST

I met with Emily Capodilupo, the director of analytics at WHOOP, whose deep background in AI powers WHOOP. The application itself provides phenomenal insights on sleep, training, and recovery, outdistancing all other training apps. Each morning after you wake up, WHOOP assesses your sleep quality, your resting heart rate, and the all-important HRV to calculate a recovery score between 0 and 100 percent. Green sparks delight with values over 66 percent! Red signaled a tough day ahead, with values below 33 percent. Yellow stood in the middle, signaling a decent but not stellar recovery, good for resilience training. WHOOP takes several weeks to calculate your baseline, then it becomes your training Bible, accurately showing you which days to crush it and which ones to dial back. After several days I was addicted and couldn't start my day until my recovery score came up. After you have settled in with your WHOOP and established a pattern, use the days you have high green recoveries for your VO2 max three-four minute intervals, your race pace intervals (anaerobic threshold, or AT), and your thirty-second neuromuscular internals. Rest assured that you will have the very greatest number of resources available to you and the least risk of injury or illness from high intensity workouts. You'll also get much better results. I've worn Garmin and other wearables for decades, but only WHOOP has the user interface, intelligent analysis, and actionable data that allow such stunning improvements to your performance! WHOOP constantly evaluates your baseline over three-day and thirty-day moving averages.

While VO2 max is a fantastic measure for your overall fitness, youth, and longevity potential, it can't be accurately measured on a daily basis. The desire for so many athletes has been to access one daily measure that shows them progress, fitness, health, and training status. HRV has come closer than any other historical measure for accomplishing this goal. Sure, resting heart rate can help and may indicate overtraining as it increases, but it simply doesn't have the accuracy or usefulness of HRV. There is simply no other barometer or measurement you can take every single day that helps so much with your training, diet, sleep, health, and recovery. Train hard on your green days, and you will boost your VO2 max. Week by week you'll be able to increase the intensity of your training in a professional training program. Your VO2 max will follow. Since HRV is so vital, let's go back to the basics.

THE HRV BASICS

HRV sits at the heart of the WHOOP device and stands for "heart rate variability." The WHOOP determines HRV by measuring the distance between each individual heartbeat on your EKG. The more variable your HRV, the springier and more elastic your body is, and therefore the better recovered and more ready your body is for a major challenge. The lower the variability in heart rate, the staler and more overtrained you are. Have a look at these two illustrations to make this clear.

Switch 1: Steady HRV: Here you can see the interval between heart rates is very steady. This is an exceedingly low heart rate variability, with very regular spaces between heartbeats.

Figure 2: Now look at a high heart rate variability—with big beat-to-beat variations. This appears far more irregular if you look closely.

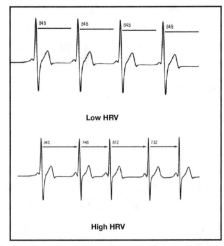

https://shonavertue.squarespace.com/vertuous-lifestyle/2018/5/15/heart

Many people think heart rate variability means how high or low your resting heart rate goes, but it doesn't. HRV measures the variation between heartbeats when you are at rest and in a deep sleep. What causes this variation? We've seen the two separate settings of your automatic nervous systems:

Switch 1: The fight-or-flight sympathetic nervous system that lights up when we are in danger, after hard a workout, or when we are overtrained. We call it sympathetic drive when the adrenalin and stress hormone areas of your nervous system increase. This drives a very low HRV score, where the beat-to-beat variation is very low, and the EKG appears quite regular. If we hammered a workout with a high fight-or flight drive, then HRV is incredibly regular, like a Swiss clock.

Switch 2: The rest-and-recovery setting calms us down and allows us to rest, sleep, and rebuild. However, if you are recovering from a strenuous workout and are really able to rest well, then HRV becomes more irregular. Why? There is less sympathetic drive to keep it regular. That means less inflammation and less aging!

WHOOP SCORES

Scores: After a month of using WHOOP, the device will establish your own highly personal green, yellow, and red zones.

Green (Clear): These are the best days you'll ever have and the best you'll feel. With big recoveries, you'll sense a peace and joy wash over you. These are the days you can feel confident in hammering your workout. You'll feel so much faster and fitter that you won't want to work out when you're not 100 percent recovered. After a long series of poor recoveries, I worked hard on all the best recovery days—and boy, did those pay off!!! I awoke on a Saturday morning with a solid 93 percent green recovery for our 2019 annual Paddle of the Bays race and took first place in the unlimited category.

Yellow Day (Gray): After a hard day, you will wake up to yellow. Back-to-back hard days will make the yellow plunge further. Professional athletes may try to build resilience by training on multiple yellow days in a row. For amateur athletes, however, two yellow days should be the max, followed by a solid green recovery.

Red Day (Black): These are the days that athletes dread, when your system has not recovered, and your sympathetic nervous system is on overdrive. There is no positive training effect on a red day, so dial it back for a very easy recovery, or take the day off. I'll just spin on an indoor exercise bike for forty minutes at a power setting of three. Red days are also a terrific barometer of sickness, injury, and overtraining, as we'll see.

For those of you who choose to measure HRV directly using your smartphone phone or a different device rather than using a WHOOP, you'll need several weeks to establish a personal high and low range and keep a daily record. I tried this with several apps but found the readings too varied to be reliable.

Q&A:

Question: If green is great, should you try to be "green" every day?

Answer: No. This means you're not getting enough stimulus. The best pattern of recoveries is jagged, with towering highs and crushing lows. People who rest all the time don't get high greens. Only by getting intense workouts and driving your HRV down can you expect it to rebound

Question: When the sympathetic nervous system is in full fight-or -flight mode, what does it do?

Answer: It dilates eyes, increases heart rate, increases the heart's force of contraction, opens up airways, dilates blood vessels in skeletal muscle to deliver more oxygen, slows down all digestive functions, and activates sweat.

Question: Does HRV have anything to do with the heart?

Answer: Not really. HRV is a very good marker for your autonomic nervous system settings.

HRV SUMMARY

HRV shows your automatic nervous system setting—stressed (Switch 1) or relaxed (Switch 2).

HRV is easily measured on a daily basis. There is simply no other marker in all of medicine that demonstrates the state of our rest and recovery better than HRV. As a lifelong fan of wearable technology, I can't overemphasize what a breakthrough the accurate daily measurement of HRV has become, showing us the daily state of our health and fitness. You require weeks between measurements of cholesterol or inflammation (C-reactive protein, or CRP, test) to see a significant change. With HRV, you can see a change the very next day.

Inexpensive yet accurate HRV measuring devices are widely available, and there are free apps for your iPhone or Android OS.

The key measures that improve our health are reflected in improved HRVs, from more exercise and sleep to losing weight, cutting calories, and smoking cessation. This allows you to do your own A/B testing to follow changes. Just keep all your other behaviors constant while you change just one, like a new diet or sleep remedy.

Relaxation efforts are also measured by increasing HRV, as I've found with yoga, better sleep, and meditation.

The decline in HRV accurately reflects how stress, lack of sleep, smoking, and alcohol or other drugs impact our health. In fact, the lowest scores are from drinking!

HRV provides for vastly superior training. HRV-guided training improved running performance (maximal running velocity) more than a pre-planned group:[30] "Pre-planned training simply refers to a program that has already been designed and does not cater for daily changes in HRV."

HRV matches VO2 max. As we'll see in the following chapter, MVO2 is the ultimate measure of youth and longevity. Researchers found that athletes who had high HRV scores improved VO2 max, whereas those who had low HRV scores showed deteriorations in VO2 max performances.[30]

DYNAMIC TRAINING PLANS

OK!!! We've looked at an exhaustive training section based on decades of the finest coaching tips. However, we have entered a new

---

30 https://www.scienceforsport.com/heart-rate-variability-hrv/

era of wearable electronic coaching that allows far greater precision and spectacular results that are unachievable without wearable tech. This is a very different and far more precise means of training. Let's take a look.

Dynamic training is vastly simpler and far more effective than traditional training, because you train hard only when your body is fresh, rested, relaxed, and has the full resources to take on a high-exercise intensity. I have suggested two stimulus days for novice and intermediate athletes and three for higher-level, competitive athletes. To recap, these are:

> Three-five-minute intervals, best for building MVO2
> Short intervals to build neuromuscular system and strength—usually 10*1 minute and 10*30 seconds
> Monday is a rest day
> For those adding a third day: twenty-thirty minutes at race pace, or substitute a competition

Look for a high HRV, high recovery, to decide which days you choose to perform these. Otherwise, dial way back to easy recovery days. It's really that simple. However, embracing HRV for your training unlocks a spectacular new world of stunning gains across all of health and fitness. You'll embrace the bright, high recovery days to crush your workouts while a new higher goal emerges ... even higher recoveries. I changed my whole philosophy of training from endless overtraining to simply trying to feel terrific. I felt better than I ever have in my entire life.

Training becomes incredibly easy. Decide on Sunday what your hard intervals are for the week, say three-minute VO2 max on one day and thirty seconds of high intensity on another. Then just wait for a high recovery day for the first one. Crush your workout. Then recover for a day or two with very easy workouts. Wait for your next high recovery day and crush it again!

Dynamic coaching allows you to apply the very strongest training stimulus to your body, since technology will tell you precisely when you are fresh, brimming with energy, fully recovered, and ready for maximal strain and benefit. This is vastly different from traditional coaching, which relies either on athlete symptoms or a stock program of easy and hard days. There's just no way to guess accurately when those days will come without technology. But with technology, you will know with great certainty when it's time to crush it. The underpinning is HRV, as we've seen. Research shows that athletes are rewarded with a higher VO2 max and faster times if they train dynamically instead of using a traditional training program based on years of trial and error.

The research: So, where's the proof that dynamic training that incorporates WHOOP or HRV works best? Several scientific studies have demonstrated the clear superiority of training based on HRV versus training based on standard coaching principles. The most encouraging proof is that VO2 max also improves more with an HRV-based program. Here are some studies that back up the research:

Study 1

This study reports superior improvement in pace and VO2 max with HRV-directed training. Twenty-six healthy, moderately fit males were randomized into two training regimens. The first group was given a predefined training program, much like you might get from a fitness magazine or a traditional coach. The second group was guided by the athlete's individual HRV measurement. Each week the traditional group ran four high-intensity and two low-intensity training sessions of forty minutes each. The HRV-guided group trained at high intensity only when there was no decrease in HRV. How did they do?

The traditional training group had only a modest increase in their training load and no increase in VO2 max. The HRV-directed group had significant increases in training load, from 15.5-16.4 kilometers/hour and VO2 max from 56-60 mg/kg. This demonstrates a stunning improvement with HRV-guided training in just four weeks.

Study 2

A pilot study in the European Journal of Sports Science[31] demonstrated that HRV was affected during exercise by the intensity and but not by duration or volume of training. Since you want highly varied HRV scores, having intense workouts is key.

Study 3

Further proof of dynamic training's superior efficiency is found in a study of cyclists. Half had a preplanned training program. The other half completed their training based on their HRV scores. Here's how they did. The HRV group improved 5 percent more at peak power, and over a forty-minute time trial, they were 7 percent faster.

Study 4

Six months of intensive aerobic exercise training increased maximum oxygen consumption by 21 percent in the older group and 17 percent in the younger group.[32] Exercise training increased HRV at rest ($p = 0.009$) by 68 percent in the older subjects and by 17 percent in the young subjects.

Study 5

A Dutch study published in the American Journal of Cardiology followed six months of training in 51 older men and women who trained for forty-five minutes, three times a week.

Studies demonstrate that regular physical activity increases HRV, while decreasing HRV is a key factor associated with an increased incidence of cardiac events.

So, let's put dynamic training into action. You'll recall from standard training that you had three intense days every week. Coaches who guessed when you should be ready for a hard day were often

31 https://www.tandfonline.com/doi/abs/10.1080/17461391.2015.1004373
32 https://www.sciencedirect.com/science/article/abs/pii/S0002914998006110

wrong, and yet had no way of knowing. Now, with dynamic training, you know with absolute certainty when you can crush your high-intensity days, and when you should lay low. So, here is how dynamic training works:

Practical application: Select your high-intensity workouts for the upcoming week. Here's an example:

High intensity, day one: 10*4 minutes
High intensity, day two: 15*1 minute, then 15*30 seconds
High intensity, day three: 6*10 minutes

When you see a green recovery day, slot the first of these workouts in. Take it easy the following day. Wait for another green recovery day, and then slot in day two. Dial back for another day or two until you see green again, then slot in the third day.

DYNAMIC TRAINING SUMMARY

Phew!!! That's a lot of complex physiology. Let's reduce this all to its innate simplicity. Your goal is undertaking the most vigorous training on the days when you bring the very most resources to your training, Here's how. Choose your intense workouts for the week, say:

10*4 minutes
15*30 seconds
20 minutes at AT

Now, wait for a high HRV or high green recovery to choose the days for these workouts.

Use SmO2 to exert the highest intensity without crossing thresholds that will risk injury or excessive fatigue. Or learn even pacing with other methods, such as speed, pace, and heart rate.

Then, between these intense workouts, enjoy a day or two of recovery at a slower and very comfortable pace. Remember that this is how Olympians train. The hardest part of training is knowing when to pull back and recover. With these astounding new tools, you can do just that.

With the new science, training is literally that simple. You'll develop tremendous insights into your own physiology and recovery over time and find a new delight in training. Why? Because you'll always feel fresh, full of energy, and ready to crush your big workouts when you are fully rested and recovered. You'll really enjoy these intense workouts. You'll see the week-by-week improvement in pace and recovery. Good luck!

Measuring success: The key is taking these decades-old, tried-and-true approaches to intensity in determining how they match up with your recovery scores. More and more, top schools like Princeton have fully embraced HRV for their athletes, training with a mix of precise biological data and traditional coaching principles. By showing that you have low recovery scores after a high-intensity day and then super-high recovery scores the following day, you know you are getting the right intensity input.

Take the case of an NBA point guard recorded at WHOOP HQ. Let's take a look at low recovery performance in a game and then high recovery:

Low recovery: 19 points a game with an average of 8 turnovers
High recovery: 22 points a game with 1 turnover

RECOVERY

I adjusted my workouts to dynamic, HRV-directed training and quickly saw benefits, with HRV moving from 28 to 45, but no higher. This was one of the greatest training revelations of my career. Why? I asked sleep expert and WHOOP Director of Analytics Emily Capodilupo. While driving HRV is a vital part of training, you can only score a super-high HRV by improving your nutrition, lowering your daily stresses, and getting more high-quality sleep. Determined to do better, I shifted my focus to everything that could affect HRV. WHOOP provides phenomenal feedback on everything you are doing—right or wrong.

What you do for the other twenty-two hours after your training determines whether or not this stimulus is effective or not. Increased quality sleep, decreased stress, and superb nutrition all create a tremendous recovery. This combination of sustained high oxygen demand in training with terrific recovery creates the very highest HRV scores.

"You think you're having a good time, but you are just a slave to something."— Mick Jagger on 60 Minutes

Mick, 76 years old as of July 2019, is staggeringly fit, but the biggest part of crushing old age was cleaning up his once abysmal rock 'n roll lifestyle!

SLEEP

Monitor your sleep. My Garmin and WHOOP devices both monitor my sleep. They make getting great sleep a contest, since sleep contributes so highly to a great recovery, a high HRV score, and overall fitness. With such great barometers, you can determine how you may have messed up, and what appears to work. My biggest insight was just how much of the night we are in a light sleep. I used to worry I was not getting enough sleep, but WHOOP showed that I did get both enough REM and deep sleep. How much of each do we need? Emily Capodilupo told me that these were fluid, and that the brain took what it needed most. I was amazed how consistently I got the same amount of deep or REM sleep, whether I slept four hours or eight. The sleep app on WHOOP is a sophisticated AI system designed by Emily, who spent seven years working at Boston's

Brigham and Women's Hospital, the second-largest teaching hospital of Harvard Medical School, with Dr. Charles Czeisler, one of the world's top academic sleep experts.

Once I observed low sleep scores and low HRV scores, I was motivated to improve my sleep like never before. Sounds crazy for zealous athletes to compete at sleeping better, but that's what I started to do. So many top athletes compare notes on sleep tips more than training! WHOOP warned me of poor sleep, then began to reward me, saying I slept better than 95 percent of WHOOP athletes. What a win. Here's what I did:

SLEEP ACTION STEPS

My sleep scores were really rocky, from 52 percent to 98 percent. Being competitive by nature, I wanted to up my sleep game to achieve much higher recovery scores. Sleep is such a huge part of recovery that I'd advise budgeting for some major bedroom upgrades. This will pay enormous dividends in how you feel and perform.

Room Preparation

Create a blacked-out room with blackout drapes and all sources of light, including night lights, hidden. You can have blackout shades custom-fit for your bedroom, or you can wear a quality eye mask.

White noise: We use an air conditioner to create white noise in the background. The best-reviewed white noise generators available on Amazon are two models from Adaptive Sound Technologies; I purchased one of them. The higher-end machine has a greater variety of sound, from nature to the conventional white, pink, and brown noise.

Sleep by a window cracked open for fresh, cold air.

Use an eye mask to blot out any extraneous light. I bought half a dozen on Amazon; my favorite were generic bean bag eye masks and a model by Brookstone.

Bose brand noise-canceling in-ear headphones. I bring these everywhere and use them just to cut the extraneous noise.

Bose noise-masking sleep buds: Bose has a new product that generates both white noise and wonderful custom sounds—tropical rain forests, birds singing, rivers flowing, and waves breaking—to play throughout the night, killing the noise of your snoring neighbor, street noises, etc. Charging them is tricky, but the devices are an ingenious advance.

Getting Ready for Bed Ritual

Take a warm shower. This is a great way to get your body ready for bed. Beginning sleep at a warmer temperature allows your body to cool, so you'll find it easier to go to sleep.

If you have a difficult time falling asleep, consider melatonin, such as Nature Made Vitamelts Fast Dissolve Melatonin. I take this, although I have no idea if it works—the research isn't convincing.

Consider yoga. I have a short yoga routine to relax before sleep.

Use blue light blocker glasses after 8 p.m. for all your screen time. The light from computers, phones, iPads, etc., has been shown to decrease your REM sleep. Check your WHOOP or Garmin sleep score to see if you don't get better REM sleep with these blockers. I increased my REM sleep by an hour with the blue light blockers. White light is like poison for sleep! You can test your glasses to see if they block white light effectively by using this URL: https://blue-blockglasses.com/blogs/news/the-rgb-color-model-test-how-effective-is-your-blue-light-filter-eyewear

Drink chamomile tea: A hot liquid helps raise body temperature so it can quickly lower as you start to fall asleep. Chamomile is a good, calming sleep inducer.

Pillows: I use Tempur-Pedic pillows and pack them with me wherever I go so I have a consistent pillow. Their form-fitting material has proven to be a miracle for great sleep!

Mattress stores have great in-house apps to test the kind of mattress you need. It's worth the investment in great sleep to have a mattress that works for you. As with my pillows, I use a Tempur-Pedic brand mattresses.

Use high-quality sheeting. You should feel great when you slide between the sheets. Great bedding makes a big difference. I suggest high-thread-count Annie Selke sheets.

Wear socks. In a very cold room, you may find your toes get icy cold. Wear a pair of socks to bed to keep the toes warm so you don't wake up with frozen feet!

Don't indulge in stressful conversations/emails before bed.

Keep to a regular bedtime schedule.

I take two SR (Sports Research) Tart Cherry Concentrate Softgels before bed.

If a protein drink will keep you awake, take the Klean-brand branched chain amino acids (BCAA) supplement when you go to bed.

Other Sleep Recommendations

Avoid alcohol, which is the great destroyer of sleep. A top college sports team saw that its recovery data did not return to normal until four days after partying! Your heart rate stays high through much of the night, until all the alcohol is out of your system. Blood alcohol should be at zero for a good night's sleep. I have a few sips of Prosecco in the early evening with my fiancé, and that's it.

Try to have your last big meal six hours or more before bedtime, and even then, eat light. A big pizza or fatty meal before bed will wreck your sleep, waking you up midway through the night, and making it hard to get back to sleep.

Get your major water consumption during the day. Try to back off after 8 p.m. so you go to sleep with an empty bladder and don't have to wake up to pee!

Drink a protein shake four hours before bedtime.

Go to bed hungry.

Take medications early if they affect sleep. For instance, certain asthma meds will elevate your heart rate. It's best to take these early in the evening.

No cheese after 6 p.m. I was shocked at how this affected my sleep. Dropping cheese decreased my awake time before falling asleep.

Stop using smartphones, tablets, computers, and gaming devices three hours before bed, and read a real book instead.

Try to go to bed at the same time every night. As WHOOP has found in its data, consistency in sleep times is the best predictor of great sleep scores.

If you toss and turn for an hour before going to sleep, go to sleep an hour later.

Get up at the same time every morning. Your body takes one hour to adjust for each hour you sleep in. So, if you get up at 6 a.m. Monday through Friday, then at 9 a.m. on Saturday, it will take you three days to recover. You'll feel like you have jet lag. If you had a late night out, get up early anyway and plan a nap.

Nap at the optimal time. This is seven hours after you get up. So, if you wake up at 7 a.m., nap at 2 p.m.[33] The optimal nap time is twenty-five minutes. If you sleep longer, you may fall into deep or REM sleep and feel groggy for hours after you get up. Take a cup of coffee before your nap, so that caffeine and napping work together to make you more alert. The caffeine won't kick in till you are up. If you nap later in the day, this may affect your ability to sleep at night. I aim for a twenty-five-minute nap at 1 p.m., which gives me a completely fresh afternoon and helps make up for any sleep deficit left over from the night.

I check my WHOOP every morning to see where I succeeded and failed. One of the most helpful observations is that we all have a lot of light sleep. If you wake up at 3 a.m., this doesn't mean you didn't have a great night's sleep. Just focus on how to get back to sleep rather than worrying about being awake. Try to have a pleasant series of thoughts. I followed this regimen, and soon I was scoring among the highest WHOOP users and had also improved my recovery scores.

---

33 https://www.sleep.org/articles/whats-the-best-time-of-the-day-to-nap/

NUTRITION

HRV is the only measure I know of that reflects the effect of nutrition on a daily basis. As an example, I had been running HRVs in the 50s with better sleep and still could not get into the 70s and 80s. Then I gave up all bread products for just one day and saw my HRV jump to 81 the following morning. The principles laid out in the nutrition section are all aimed at improving HRV. As Will Ahmed told me, WHOOP gives you the ideal way to do your own A/B testing. That is, try one diet and then another to observe the change in HRV. Scientists experimented with rabbits and found that a high-fat, high-sugar diet showed a 54 percent drop in heart rate variability.[34] Here are other effects of nutrition on HRV in this study:

Decreased HRV:
High intakes of saturated or trans fat
High glycemic carbohydrates,[35] e.g., white bread
Skipping breakfast (true for humans as well)

Action Steps: Part II, the section on fuel, has it all!!!

MENTAL HEALTH

Depressed? Anxious? Depression throws us into a tailspin physically. Our rest-and-recovery nervous system is thrown into disarray, and when that happens, HRV plummets.

HRV has proven itself to be a powerful tool in lifting the veil of depression. Using HRV as a barometer of mental health, patients have been able to improve sleep, lower levels of stress, and improve HRV as a result.

Research:[36] The lower HRV found in depressed patients may

---

34 https://www.ncbi.nlm.nih.gov/pubmed/31426570
35 https://www.dovepress.com/heart-rate-variability-measurement-and-clinical-depression-in-acute-co-peer-reviewed-fulltext-article-ND
36 https://www.ncbi.nlm.nih.gov/pubmed/29543648

explain a high degree of sympathetic dysfunction and hence an increased risk of heart attack.

Research demonstrates that treating depression with cognitive behavioral therapy may reduce heart rate and increase short-term HRV. The study concluded that CBT "... may have a beneficial effect on a risk factor for mortality in depressed patients with coronary heart disease."[37]

MEDITATION

Many professional WHOOP users rely on meditation to reduce stress. I meditate while doing my evening Bikram Yoga routine. You may try the fabulous app Headspace, which walks your through inspiring meditation sessions. You'll feel a wave of calm come over you as you end each session. Professional athletes spend a great deal of time and effort on cutting the distractions around them.

REDUCING THE RISK OF HEART DISEASE[38]

Study: A low HRV has been associated with a higher incidence of cardiac events and total mortality. Most older individuals have both a higher risk of cardiac events and a low amount of physical activity. This study in the journal Medicine and Science in Sports and Exercise looked at the effect of six months of physical training in a group of fifty-one older women and men. They just trained forty-five minutes, three times a week.

Result: This study demonstrated that regular physical activity increases HRV. The authors concluded: "In older subjects, physical training may be an effective means to modify positively a factor that is associated with increased incidence of cardiac events."

---

37 https://journals.lww.com/psychosomaticmedicine/Abstract/2000/09000/Change_in_Heart_Rate_and_Heart_Rate_Variability.7.aspx
38 https://europepmc.org/abstract/med/10378908

ATRIAL FIBRILLATION:
THE MASTER'S GREATEST FEAR

"Bob! Look at this!" On the bus from the Oslo airport to the World Masters Nordic Championships, Dave, a seasoned Nordic ski racer, showed me a paper on the risk of atrial fibrillation (AF) in Master athletes with a look of deep concern on his face. This heart condition is the dreaded scourge of aging endurance athletes. The longer you train, the higher your risk. This gives some older athletes serious second thoughts about continuing to train hard. Atrial fibrillation signifies a wildly irregular rhythm in your heart's auxiliary pump, the atrium. AF decreases your effective cardiac output and puts you at risk for stroke. You'll be put on meds to thin your blood (anticoagulants) and to help control your heart rate or rhythm. There is a technique to cut the pathways in the pulmonary veins that generate AF. I would advise having this procedure as soon as your doctor will allow, if your AF is becoming chronic.

So, against this backdrop, most older athletes would welcome a way to prevent atrial fibrillation. While I do not have a panacea, HRV may prove very useful. Here's why. A low HRV increases your risk of AF. There are three potential reasons for this:

1. You never let your body recover, so you are under constant strain.
2. You have poor nutrition and a poor lifestyle, which lowers HRV and increases your risk of AF.
3. The constant high sympathetic activity in your automatic nervous system stresses the atria.

Now, here's how WHOOP/HRV can help lower your risk of AF, increasing HRV:

1. Try to get a green day after every yellow or red day of training by training hard on green days, backing off on yellow days, and resting on red days.

2. Improve your nutrition and tremendously decrease your inflammation by following the program in the chapter on fuel.

3. Improve your sleep, using the WHOOP sleep coach.

4. Improve your overall health by working with your MD on stress, blood pressure, cholesterol, body weight, and other key measures of health. Doctors focus first on these measures of health in a patient newly diagnosed with AF. Many times, the frequency of AF diminishes with improved health. These steps may help you lower the risk of AF by raising your HRV. I'm just as fearful of AF as any older athlete and carefully follow my own advice! My HRV had been as low as 28. Now I'm usually in the seventies on a green day and have hit 115.

CHAPTER 8

THE FULL RESTORATION OF YOUTH

OK!!! Let's put it all together! After plowing through some tough science, here is the reward as promised: Finally flipping the youth switch! At the beginning of this book, we looked at how researchers selected HRV as the ultimate marker for the full restoration of youth. Here's what they said:

"It is well established that HRV is a measure of biological age. Biological age correlates heavily with homeostatic capacity, which is the body's ability to self-stabilize in response to stressors. Studies have shown that biological age is a better measure for determining health status and risk than chronological age."[39]

Find your HRV? Now let's look at your actual HRV values for your age and sex.

The journal Frontiers in Physiology published a paper entitled, "Normal Value of Corrected HRV in 10-second Electrocardiograms

39 https://hrvcourse.com/hrv-demographics-age-gender/

for All Ages."[40] The article reported the first comprehensive set of normal values for heart-rate-corrected, ten-second HRV (the unit measured as RMSSD, or Root Mean Square of the Successive Differences, which is the standard used by WHOOP and many other devices.)

Age	Male	Female
1-2	141	150
3-4	131	138
5-7	118	126
8-11	102	109
12-15	84	93
16-19	70	80
20-29	51	63
30-39	37	47
40-49	29	35
50-59	24	27
60-69	20	22
70-79	19	20
80-89	17	19

Let's look at the data. You can see spectacular scores in youth well over 100, then averaging in the seventies for teenagers, and declining each decade after the teens into your eighties, when women average 19 and men 17. Really low. Check your own HRV against your age.

Women and HRV

The study "Short-Term Heart Rate Variability—Influence of Gender and Age in Healthy Subjects," by Voss A et al. (2015) reported that males typically have lower HRV than females within the same age ranges. This indicates that males exhibit stronger sympathetic (fight-or-flight stress response) drive than comparable females.[41] That may be why women are on a more even keel than men and live longer! Spectacular HRVs at every age.

40 https://www.frontiersin.org/articles/10.3389/fphys.2018.00424/full
41 The study "Short-Term Heart Rate Variability—Influence of Gender and Age in Healthy Subjects," by Voss A et al. (2015) shows that males typically have lower Heart Rate Variability than females within the same age ranges. This indicates that males exhibit stronger Sympathetic (fight-or-flight stress response) tendencies over Parasympathetic (rest-and-digest) than comparable females.

The Journey

My first HRV reading was a depressing 28 and perilously close to the value for my real age group. Ouch!!! To up my HRV score, I radically changed my training program, trying to get a huge aerobic boost from my workouts, then get solid rest and recovery following the principles of dynamic training. After a month, my HRV moved into the fifties, what you would expect for a 25-year-old. However, I wanted to push the Palo Alto Foundation thesis to the limit and see if I could do far better. As they say, you spend one-two hours training a day, but it's what you do in the other twenty-two to twenty-three hours that count most. I hired a nutrition consultant to up my nutrition game. QT2 Systems put me in touch with Rachel Gargano. She took a careful dietary history and then drastically improved what I ate, cutting out all junk carbs and adding a range of super-nutrients. Nutrition brought my scores further up into the sixties. Finally, I turned to sleep, using every technique I could unearth to improve, as discussed in the previous chapter. Tons to improve! As collegiate and professional athletes encounter low HRV scores, they become extremely competitive about sleep so that they can hit the

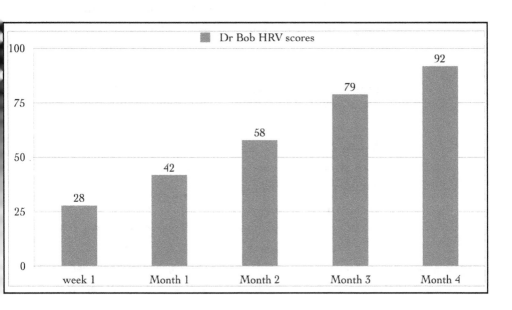

very highest HRV and recovery scores. Finally, a solid focus on sleep brought my average HRV into the seventies with spikes as high as 131. Magic! The results would astonish the prize committee. Have a look. I was both astounded and incredibly pleased at how high my HRV climbed, and how amazing I felt.

Now let's look at this step by step. What I love best about HRV is that you're rewarded every day and every week with observable progress, as you start to see better and better recoveries and watch your HRV climb. You know that as it climbs and as your pace improves, your MVO2 is improving as well.

> **Step 1:** Select an activity that you love that develops a large VO2 max.
>
> **Step 2:** Gradually increase the volume of exercise you can do an hour or more a day.
>
> **Step 3:** Begin to focus on rest by taking Mondays off.
>
> **Step 4:** Introduce three-five-minute intervals once a week followed by a day of light activity. Begin with 4*3–minute intervals. Increase so you can perform eight to ten three-minute intervals. Then increase the length of your intervals to four minutes after several months. Finally, increase these intervals to five minutes in length. Keep your speed and heart rate constant, so that you are getting a great aerobic load throughout the full interval. SmO2 devices are of the most benefit here, ensuring a consistent load. The biggest mistake here is to go all out in the first fifteen seconds and then spend the rest of the interval recovering
>
> **Step 5:** Add a second day of thirty-second intervals. Build so you can do ten of these. Take enough time in between to rest and let your heart rate and SmO2 recover.
>
> **Step 6:** Finally, if you compete or are trying to do well at charity rides or fun runs, add a day at race pace. This would be the speed you can hold steadily for twenty-five minutes and should be close to your anaerobic threshold. You should be comfortably winded. Training at this pace lends you a much higher usage of your total

VO2 max and gives you your best speed advantage.

Step 7: Begin focusing on improvements in your nutrition, as outlined in the Fuel section of this book.

Step 8: Amass as many sleep tools as possible to vastly improve the quality of your sleep, following the sleep guidelines in this book.

Step 9: Finally, look at all the resources you are spending unnecessarily on the stress in your life. Embrace a meditation strategy such as Headspace.

As you undertake these steps, watch the steady improvement in HRV and recovery scores with great satisfaction.

Timeline

Week 1: Expect your first changes in HRV.

Month 1: Expect to move from your age group to a younger one with exercise.

Month 2: Expect to move toward real youth with improvements in nutrition.

Month 3: Expect to have your sleep scores increase even more.

Month 4: With a more relaxed lifestyle and lower stress, expect scores of healthy individuals in their twenties.

Recovery

Reward is the most powerful incentive to any kind of lifestyle change. As you embrace a training with vigorous interval days followed by easy recovery days and rest, you'll see your recovery scores soar within a week or two of beginning. If you're a Groundhog Day athlete, with a dull repetitive program day in and out, you will be astonished both by how well you feel and by the incredible recovery scores you'll attain by changing to this program. Just introduce two high-intensity interval days, a rest day, and low intensity for the remainder. I was totally fried from the World Master Nordic Championships. Within a week, I was getting these astonishing recovery scores—just by introducing this mix of rest, low intensity, and high intensity.

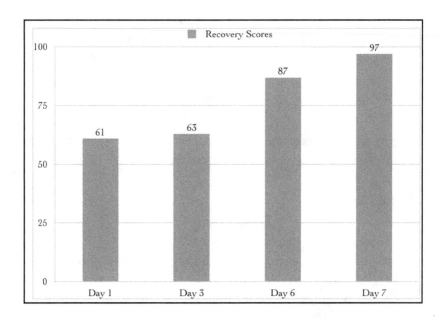

WHOOP combines sleep, resting heart rate (RHR), and HRV to come up with its overall recovery score. RHR can be a great measure of fitness and health, and it is a point of pride among athletes. RHR is both a great overall barometer of fitness and a terrific day-to-day value. My best is 39 beats per minute, but with stress and over-training, it will drift up to 55 BPM.

Risk of a high resting heart rate: The journal Heart[42] followed 3,000 men for sixteen years. The study reported that a high resting heart rate was linked to:

Higher blood lipids (cholesterol, triglycerides)
Higher blood pressure
Higher body weight
Poor physical fitness
A higher risk of premature death

42 https://www.sciencedaily.com/releases/2013/04/130415204911.htm

The authors calculated that every ten to twenty-two additional beats per minute in resting heart rate increased the risk of death by 16 percent overall. So, if your resting heart rate is 90, your risk of death has tripled! Good reasons to get it down! As your RHR drops, it's a direct indication that your VO2 max is increasing! RHR is best measured first thing in the morning, before you get out of bed. WHOOP will measure automatically during deep sleep.

Q&A:

Question: Can I just get high green scores by resting and relaxing all the time?

Answer: Great idea!!! However, this does not work. You cannot generate the highest green recoveries and HRV scores without high-intensity aerobic workloads.

Question: Can I get the highest HRV scores playing racket sports, working out in the gym, or weight lifting?

Answer: No. The evidence is that the aerobic athletes get the very highest score. The best workaround is to have a training sport like cycling or hill climbing, where you get two intense aerobic interval workouts a week in addition to your gym routine, racket sports, and weight training.

CHAPTER 9

HOW TO CHOOSE YOUR MOST SUCCESSFUL SPORT

Each of us has tremendous natural gifts that allow us to be great at a specific sport. Some of us may have found those as a high school or college athlete. But chances are that most of us have simply fallen into a convenient fitness activity that fits into our schedule and is easily available, like running or walking. However, running, as an example, is a sport we are unlikely to be widely successful at unless we have a highly specific body type. Marathon runners have a very lean body type, weighing just two pounds per inch of body weight. I weighed 200 pounds at 6'4". I'd have to weigh an unimaginably light 152 pounds. Marathoners add long legs, narrow hips, a high MVO2, and a pre-dominance of endurance muscle fiber type. Like so many, I blundered ahead and built a running career, competing in scores of 10K, 10-mile, triathlon, marathon, and finally Ironman competitions. On the inbound leg of the marathon portion of the Cape Cod Endurance Triathlon, I noticed my hips felt strange. X-rays showed that I had worn away nearly all of the cartilage in my hips. I eventually had hip surgery, but I suffered for many years afterward. I'm a prime example of someone choosing a highly popular sport without realizing it wasn't for me! Running destroyed my hips.

As you hit huge milestones—40, 50, and 60—I'd ask you to reconsider your sports. Why? First, there is an incredible adventure in store for you with new fitness activities. Find something you truly love. With a lifelong passion for surfing, I chose long-distance, big-wave, stand-up surfing. This incorporated all I had ever done:

The balance of surfing
The endurance of the Ironman
The power of rowing
The agility of ski racing
The pack racing tactics of cycling
The aerobic challenge of Nordic skiing

If you don't already have these talents, you'll have an amazing time developing them. I'm a lifelong student of motor learning, a lesser-known part of exercise science. Few of us realize that we can learn brand new sports later in life and excel at them. I went from falling off a board twenty-five times in my first race at the Pacific Paddle Games to winning the world championship twice in my age group for SUP.

So, consider several factors:

What are you really good at?
What would you like to be really good at?
What makes a sport a play sport for you?

Let's look at several scenarios:

1. You're a lifelong runner and want to stick with it. Sure. If you have a lightweight frame, are highly competitive, and injury-free, you could continue running for a lifetime. You will lose muscle elasticity,

which will slow you down, and you risk a large loss of muscle mass in your seventies and eighties. You could add cycling to improve elasticity and drive your heart and lungs. You could also take the enormous heart-lung power you have developed and harness it to a new activity, like SUP, surfski, Nordic skiing, or rowing, where there's no pounding, and you would gain a tremendous ability to maintain your VO2 max. If you stick with running, dynamic training will allow you to make much larger gains and also avoid overtraining and injury.

2. You're a jogger, but you are slowing down and developing joint aches and pains. OK. You are an ideal candidate to add a new sport to drive your fitness. Your forties and fifties are the ideal time to transition. You'll dramatically increase your fitness and athleticism.

3. You're a lifelong cyclist. Keep it up! You can cycle into your nineties and maintain a fanatic MVO2. You'll get much more out of your workouts with dynamic training and using the latest electronic gear, which measures power output, SmO2, and HRV.

4. You're just starting a serious fitness program and want a sport that helps you recreate youth. Great! Find something you love. Just don't be intimidated into thinking you can't learn. You can learn, and you can become incredibly great! I've seen this with dozens of athletes I've brought into SUP. You'll be able to determine what you can do best. Focus on the sports that are best at building and maintaining a high VO2 max, as we saw in the first part of this book.

How to Get Good

So, I hope you're sold on exploring new activities and embracing new, more technical, sports like SUP and cross-country skiing. But how? The answer is found in two incredibly powerful areas of sports science that we'll have a look at now: motor learning[43]—or how to best learn new sports and biomechanics—and how to technically perfect your new activity. If you have young children, you'll love learning how they learn best!

---

43 Imaging in Movement Disorders: Imaging Methodology and Applications in Parkinson's Disease Massimo Filippi, ... Federica Agosta, in International Review of Neurobiology, 2018

HOW TO LEARN A NEW SPORT

Part 1: Motor Learning

In looking through the amazing options in sports and activities that can boost your VO2 max and start your journey toward the restoration of youth, you may balk and say, "Not for me." One significant reason why so many adults resist is that they have a poor motor literacy that is left over from childhood, where they either hyper-focused on one sport or just didn't get a wide-enough exposure to a variety of sports and activities, from gymnastics and soccer to wall-climbing and hiking, As a result, they don't feel they have the motor coordination to begin Nordic skiing, rowing, or cycling, I tell any good runners that they can harness stunning heart and lung power to more technical sports that will soften the blow on their joints and allow them to excel once again. This all comes down to having the confidence that you can learn and excel in any sport you choose—with careful coaching and practice. I was a terrible childhood athlete, but I've been able to master half a dozen sports as an adult—and you can to. How do I know? From my experience and research in the field of motor learning. In World War II, those aviators who had a lot of error correction practice actually became safer, better aviators than the aviators who were natural athletes. So, by learning great form, you too may exceed the performance of the natural athlete, through practice and persistence. Not only can you get good at sports that are brand new to you, but you can also win! When I coach soccer, the natural athletes will learn a new drill with two tries. The most untalented will learn in five tries. As a coach, I stick with that athlete for the full five tries. That way, they score a big win—and as a result, the whole team wins.

Theory: Harvard's Howard Gardner described seven different kinds of intelligence. One of them is Bodily-Kinesthetic Intelligence ("body smart"), or how well we are able to use our bodies to solve problems, employing mental skills and abilities to coordinate how our bodies perform in sports, dance, and other skilled activities. Gardner sees mental and physical activity as related. If you're plummeting down a steep slope in fresh, deep snow and suddenly see a large tree trunk in your path, this is a problem you can't sit down and figure out with a calculator—you have to figure this out in a split-second. Life or death stuff! This real-time problem-solving is a constant intellectual challenge. I'm always thinking about how to improve a stroke at paddle boarding, a backhand in tennis, a skate movement in Nordic skiing, a "step turn" in skin mountaineering racing, or an arc in giant slalom (GS) racing. This makes fitness both a mental challenge and real fun, while keeping your interest level high—like a real-life video gamer! Many of us plod along in a non-skill sport, when we could undertake a real intellectual challenge and improve our fitness in many ways at the same time. Take SUP, which combines the skills of Nordic skiing, snowboarding, surfing, and bike racing. Every day I work out, I learn something new.

Exercise scientists study how we acquire new skills by learning, then refining, them. There are three main phases of motor learning. Too many of us believe in the myth of the natural athlete, who steps into a sport already an expert and star. This has discouraged generations of would-be athletes, who falsely believe they are too uncoordinated or lack enough talent to succeed. Nothing could be further from the truth. I am not a natural athlete. At summer camp, I was put in left field with another left fielder, just in case a ball ever came in my direction. I'm a completely self-developed athlete with no apparent natural skill or ability. But by understanding motor learning and continuing to practice and refine, I've acquired a myriad of highly satisfying skills that have gotten me to many world championships. Your key is error correction. Flail around, try your best, look like an idiot. Then learn to adapt from great coaches, whose vision allows them to quickly diagnose and correct your errors. Yes, finding that coach may be a challenge. Most coaches are unconsciously competent, or they may be able to show you what to do, but they are unable to diagnose your flaws and correct them while refining your technique. An average tennis coach my take years to improve your game. Then there are coaches like those at Nick Bolletieri's IMG Tennis Academy in Florida or Topnotch Tennis Academy in Vermont. These top pros could instantly diagnose all my flaws in twenty minutes, then send me off with remedial drills.

I encourage you to believe in yourself and your ability to acquire and refine skills that will give you a new horizon in terms of sports activities and challenges. The key is understanding the process of motor learning. Here's a brief synopsis.

Phase 1: Cognitive: You'll learn about a new sport through four key inputs: understanding, seeing, feeling, and doing. Your performance will be highly erratic but will improve with good coaching. The key is to learn what coaching cues work best for you. Anyone at this stage is going to look uncoordinated, unskilled, and clueless. Don't be embarrassed; don't quit. Everyone goes through this early stage. If you have kids, encourage them to understand that they will feel frustrated, even hopeless, at the beginning, but they will gradually improve. My 7-year-old could only hit the tennis ball if it were rolled toward him on the ground, and even then, he might miss. But through steady practice, he could hit it at the net, then halfway back, and finally from the baseline. What worked was giving him the confidence to succeed. Early learning is all about refining movements through good coaching and error correction. This phase requires a huge amount of attention from your brain, and it will totally consume you. This can become overwhelming. I skied with fifty-two different directives I was working on! Your frontal and parietal lobes of your brain are at full activity, requiring all your attention.

Phase 2: Associative: You consolidate all the instruction into more coordinated movements as your skills become refined, your shots more accurate, and your error rate lower. This still requires lots of mental effort, but you'll begin to feel confident!

Phase 3: Autonomous:[44] In the early cognitive phase, your entire brain lit up, and the effort seemed overwhelming. During the final autonomous phase, your movements become more and more au-

---

44 Marinelli et al., 2017

tomatic. You don't even think about them. This requires much less of your brain's concentration. I think of motor learning like writing a computer program or learning a new language. Once all the pieces are put together, the program executes flawlessly/you speak fluently. You'll feel fluid and be able to react to your environment, whether that is a squash court or surfboard. In fact, think of beginning surfers as they stumble to get up on their board during practice. Eventually the move becomes so automatic that they flawlessly pop up on their board and then execute incredible turns down the wave, then back up the wave, and into the air! You'll look like a natural athlete. I tell friends I'm a totally constructed, artificial athlete, in the sense that I've just mastered motor learning, even though I have few innate skills.

Application: Understand how you learn best and then acquire the skills you need to explore a world of amazing new sports. Don't be limited by what you know from the past. Learn to stand-up paddle, play tennis, row, and/or ski mountaineer. Take the challenge .Try new sports that provide tremendous leverage on your cardiovascular system.

HOW TO LEARN A NEW SPORT

Part 2: Biomechanics

Proper biomechanics allow you to load your muscles much more vigorously, enjoy a far better workout, and prevent injury while learning flawless technique.

In my winter sports lab in Lake Placid, we had a visiting professor, Chuck Dillman, a genius at biomechanics. He observed ski jumping. The American jumpers uncoiled, unbending their knees at a rate of less than 300 degrees per second. By contrast, the world's best jumpers registered more than 400 degrees. If US ski jumpers could recognize this slow angular velocity when unbending their knees, he instructed, those jumpers could learn to improve their speed at takeoff. Top jumpers applied the newer, higher angular velocity technique, and they went from the bottom of the pack to the top. Understanding the mechanics of your sport will dramatically improve your skill and performance.

I've chosen SUP as a demonstration sport. Have a look, even if you have no intention of learning the sport, to get a sense of the exquisite detail and of the specific cues that should be developed to improve in any sport. In SUP, many beginners overuse their arms and hinge at the waist, developing tremendous lower back, shoulder, and trapezius pain. With the right biomechanics, beginners learn to use their body weight for maximum leverage, dropping onto their paddle and using all the core muscles to propel themselves. Every single day I paddle, ski, or Nordic ski, I learn something completely new. This makes each of my workouts much more enjoyable, plus I have the satisfaction of improving every day. Choosing technically complex sports are especially rewarding, since you learn something new and improve your technique during every single workout. Since stand-up paddleboards are so universally available, rent one for an hour or two and try this out. Once you master motor learning in one sport, you can much more easily apply it to them all! The key is to understand where the power is coming from, and then how all of the power levers are pulled together into one fluid stroke! Read through the following and paint a mental picture of how you would SUP, even if you aren't going to become a SUP athlete. This is great practice!

SUP: THE LEVERS OF POWER

Many paddlers think of how good their stroke looks, wanting a pretty or elegant stroke instead of a fast, powerful stroke. That's a big mistake. You want to look at how you are generating power and maximize each of these core power generators. Where does the power come from? Let's take a look at power generators:

Weight drop: Dropping your body weight suddenly and decisively at the beginning of the stroke generates the most power. Then dropping your hips down and back continues the power generation.

Hip torque: Borrowing a technique from athletes who race C1 canoes, torqueing—or twisting the hips—generates significant power on the blade. By reaching far forward and pressing your paddle-side hip, hand, knee, and shoulder far forward, you maximize your potential hip torque.

Abdominals: Your abdominals should be fully stretched before each stroke to pre-load them for a vigorous contraction. As soon as your paddle engages the water at the catch, your abdominals engage. Contract them as hard as you can to force the paddle through the water while pressing your top hand down on the blade.

Pressing hips back: Once your paddle is fully seated, you can generate huge amounts of power by dropping your hips down, or down and back, as you press on the top of the paddle with your latissimus dorsi muscles, or lats.

Lats press-down: Pressing down on the top of the paddle with your lats adds significant extra power. The greatest added power is the torquing and twisting your shoulders, with lots of added lats power. You'll feel a highly satisfactory engagement in the lats as they engage with the paddle. The biomechanical cue is to feel the top of your upper lat engage and then feel the muscle contract down its whole length as you finish your stroke.

Forward catapult: This is the fastest and most powerful part of the strokes of SUP champions Connor Baxter and Dave Kalama, yet it is widely ignored by most paddlers. This catapult uses all of your leg muscles and lats to return your body to a ready position for the beginning of the new stroke. Connor does this as an ankle snap in sprints. For longer distances, you'll see the best paddlers keep their paddle in the water, under significant pressure, as they bring their hips forward into the start position for a new stroke.

Stroke Phases

Preparation: As your body weight launches forward at the end of the stroke, take a split second to position your body precisely for the attack, making sure your blade is as far forward as possible, your lower arm is forward and pulling out of the socket, and your hips are fully twisted forward on the side of your stroke and ready to uncoil. Steady your board with your feet so that it is completely balanced in the water.

Attack: Drop your paddle and body weight toward the water with great velocity and acceleration. Your paddle should enter the water clean and fast. Why? Because you want to engage your entire body in pulling on the paddle as soon as possible. Even a delay of a few hundred milliseconds will lose you a foot or more of blade travel and huge amounts of power. Connor Baxter has the most aggressive attack, holding his blade well off the water and dropping his entire body weight quickly, then allowing the blade to enter the water as his downward weight drop reaches its highest velocity.

Slice: Your paddle should slice cleanly into the water, with no splash at all. The paddle should enter at great velocity, so that it is seated for the pull to begin. You can lose a foot to eighteen inches of blade travel if you enter slowly, splash as you enter, or don't keep enough downward pressure on the handle. Try to feel no effort in your back or arms as you silently slide your paddle deep into the water.

Catch: The most vital power preparation in paddling is burying your blade in the water with a highly positive angle. This serves as the anchor for your stroke. So vital is the catch to paddling that the famous coach Johnny Puakea spent a full year improving his catch.

Cues

Feel: The paddle should feel like it is stuck in concrete once it is fully seated in the water, and it should move through the water with tremendous difficulty. That's because you are actually pulling your board to the paddle, and you are not pulling your paddle through the water. Most of us mistake paddling with pulling the blade through the water. If you can pull the paddle through the water, it means the paddle is too shallow, and you are cheating the stroke.

Visual cue: Look down at your blade. If you see a whirlpool effect, water movement, or a splash around the blade, then you have lost your grip on the water.

Entry mark: Look for a mark far forward on your board where you slice your paddle into the water. For instance, on a starboard, you may want to aim for the "S". See how far back on the board your paddle is before it is fully seated and engages.

Lower arm: Roll your lower arm forward, so it feels like it is coming forward out of its socket and extend your arm and hand as far as possible toward the front of your board. With your upper hand behind, this sets up the forward blade angle. Punch forward and down with your lower hand as you are recovering at the end of the stroke to get the paddle as far forward as possible.

Reach, reach, reach!!!

Errors

Most paddlers lower their paddle toward the water even as they already begin to bring the paddle backward along the board. As the paddle hits the water in this scenario, it splashes, does not fully enter the water, and does not exert full power until halfway through the stroke—the cause of many sore shoulders and backs!

Most paddlers suffer a huge amount of slippage as their blade begins its journey through the water due to poor paddle seating, a negative blade angle, and a catch that is too far back. This results in a tremendous loss of power and speed.

In a race, I find that just reaching further forward and planting solidly improves my speed immediately.

Drive: With your blade solidly anchored, you can exert maximum force to accelerate board travel by pressing firmly on the top of the paddle with your lats as your body uncoils and pulls the paddle backward. Your body weight continues the acceleration, and you prepare to catapult in one continuous motion.

Catapult: This is the most poorly understood and executed part of the stroke. Connor Baxter does it best. Larry Cain's theory is that if you pull your paddle out of the water and recover at the end of the stroke, you are pushing your board backward and losing speed. Larry advocates leaving the blade in the water as you move your body weight forward. However, you can accelerate your board dynamically by pulling yourself forward with your lower hand as you snap your ankles to propel your body mass forward. This is incredibly elegant when done properly. It's also fantastic for launching yourself onto waves during a downwind. Some boards, such as Starboard's Ace, Allstar, and Sprint models, have built-in features that allow you to flex and propel them forward. This is the extra edge you can use to win a race. This dynamic leg drive is the future of the sport, since this allows you to engage your biggest muscles and a larger percentage of your maximal oxygen uptake.

Paddle velocity: As your paddle strikes the water, it should be moving extremely slowly through it if it is properly locked and seated in the water. Then accelerate the blade right to the end of the stroke as you bring maximum leverage, coming to a hard stop at the end of the stroke as you then launch your body weight forward with a solidly planted blade. You should be accelerating throughout the stroke, reaching the highest force at the very end, after which you should feel your board go into a glide phase and its greatest forward speed.

Steadying: This last phase of the stroke is vital in tough ocean conditions, choppy water, and downwinds. This is a momentary pause to adjust your balance and completely relax your muscles as you stand fully recovered, with your hips forward and ready to begin a new stroke. I learned this from Dave Kalama when the wave faces at Ho'okipa were thirty feet tall one brutal January as we paddled from Maliko Gulch to Kahului Harbor.

Balance: Many beginning SUP athletes try to balance by pushing their feet down on either side of the board. This leads to a violent rocking back and forth, until the athlete enters the water headfirst! Vastly preferred is moving your hips laterally—from left to right and right to left—to adjust your balance while keeping your feet still and the board completely flat. If you snap your ankles at the end of the stroke to launch yourself forward, you will balance the board. As you are slightly airborne, you will have a chance to regain your balance.

INDIVIDUAL BODY PARTS

As you improve, you will want to focus on each key body part to perfect your stroke, decrease your likelihood of injury, and improve your power.

Wrist: Your lower arm and hand should form a straight line, with your wrist breaking neither up nor down.

Cues

Look at your wrist at the beginning of each stroke and determine that there is no angle between your arm and wrist. The line along your forearm and onto your wrist should be completely flat. Your wrist should not break up or down.

Error

Many paddlers break their wrist downward, which causes them to "top" the paddle blade; that is, add too much power pressing forward on the top of the paddle blade instead of pulling the paddle with the bottom arm. This causes the paddle to go into a negative blade angle, substantially decreasing power, even though it may feel fast. This gives you less reach and puts more strain on the triceps and weaker muscle groups—one reason why paddlers get sore muscles.

Grip: Top hand: Your grip should be extremely light. The palm of your hand should gently rest on top of the paddle handle, with your fingers loosely dropping over the top and not gripping the paddle. Gripping the paddle and breaking your wrist downward "tops" the paddle with a negative blade angle. You should be able to leave your hand open and loose, with the pressure right in the middle of your hand next to the meaty part.

Bottom hand: Connor Baxter, World Champion, advocates loosely gripping the paddle with just two fingers.

Errors

A death grip increases muscle tension and will cause rapid fatigue. As you press your upper hand down on the paddle handle, your elbow should be neutral, neither pointing up to the sky nor down toward the water. This allows you to get the greatest amount of leverage on the top of your paddle by using your largest back muscles, the lats. I like to start with my hand high and close to my head, so that I get the greatest blade angle.

Pointing your elbow down, the weaker triceps muscles and increases strain and the likelihood of fatigue.

Pointing your elbow up lacks power.

Your lower arm should act as a solid, passive link between your paddle and your body; it should be completely straight. As you drop your weight down and back, it is your lower arm that is pulling the blade through the water. Any bend in your elbow introduces a weak link, fatigue, and possible injury. You may pull hard at the very end of the strike.

Bent elbow: Muscling through the stroke by progressively bending your elbow like a biceps curl in the gym is an error. Your core strength and body weight add infinitely more power than the small biceps.

Tight grip: Your hips are the greatest power levers in the sport. Your paddle-side hip should be as far forward of your opposite hip as comfortable. This puts your paddle as far forward as possible and provides the biggest opportunity to generate torque as your stroke begins.

Paddle-side hip should be neutral.

Both hips should be flexed rather than extended, losing stored kinetic energy for the stroke.

Hips throughout the stroke:

Begin: Move your hips as far forward as you can, with your paddle-side hip leading as much as is comfortable. The distance your hip can travel down and back determines most of the blade travel and power, so you want to create the greatest potential range.

Middle: Drive your hips down and back, or directly down. I mix it up during long races, using both techniques.

End: Drive your hips forward again by snapping your ankles and squeezing your buttocks while pulling yourself forward with your bottom hand with the paddle still in the water. Most paddlers miss this part: they pull the paddle out during recovery and lose the biggest lever of power.

Unilateral: Top canoeists like Larry Cain and Tommy Buday drive with just the paddle-side hip rather than both hips.

Knees: Comfortably bend your knees in an athletic stance, as if you were skiing. Your knees should be over your feet for added stability. Stand duck-footed to accentuate this.

An "A" frame with your legs forming the upper part of the A is another error.

Blade: A positive blade angle means that your paddle has an angle greater than straight up and down; that is, your bottom hand and blade are forward of your upper hand and handle. You should look at the blade before it enters the water to determine its position. Many paddlers begin with no angle at all and then push back really hard way past their feet. This negative bad angle drives the board down into the water and actually slows it down. The blade should stay in as positive an angle as possible during the stroke. Once your blade starts to go negative, end your stroke, since you are pushing your board down into the water and slowing down.

Another error is beginning your stroke with a natural or negative blade angle.

Yet another error is continuing your stroke past your feet when the blade angle is positive. Your feet are ultimately what push the board forward through the water.

Cue

Feel the balls of your feet push your board forward as your hips drop back. At the end of your rear hip drive, as you dig your paddle in hard and begin to drive your hips forward, you will be pushing your board forward with your feet. You will do this both by snapping your ankles to propel your body weight up and forward and squeezing your buttocks. At the end of the recovery, stand up on the balls of your feet if you can.

Example: I ran the Onion River Race and Scramble on the Winooski River in Vermont this year, always trying to eke out a bit more speed. I found that if I just stuck the paddle in the water and pushed the board forward with my feet, I could get 0.2 mph, which is a huge amount. I also felt the pressure on the outside of my feet, so that I brought my knees over the top of my feet.

Practice each power lever until it is perfected. Then you can link all of them together into a fluid stroke. Remember, making a motor program for sports is like learning a language. First you need to learn the words. Those are the small motor programs. Then you link them into a full sentence for a full motor program—the stroke.

The usable stroke: Your GPS speedometers will indicate that you may generate tremendous speed for thirty seconds, perhaps over 7 mph, but what top speed can you make for an hour? You may find that your shoulder muscles or triceps tire quickly. That's why coaches like Larry Cain focus on a usable stroke, where no one muscle group is over-taxed. I like to have at least two different strokes, so I can mix them up. I also like to be able to generate more power with my legs into a steep headwind, and more with my upper body to rest my legs on a downwind. Legs are more resistant to fatigue.

METRICS

How do you know if these power levers are working? A GPS device with a very fast refresh displaying almost instantaneous speed is best. I work on one power lever at a time and look at the effect on speed. SUP-specific devices like the new Velocitek Makai display speed updated multiple times per second to reflect the effect of a single stroke. I have my board set up like a race car, with the following measurements:

Heart rate

Speed

Stroke rate

Distance per stroke

SmO2

As a physician and exercise scientist, this helps me in innumerable ways. I watch my gauge throughout all workouts and races. I set up my Nordic skis and bicycles with a similar dashboard.

Again, while you might not aspire to be a paddler, do read through this section and imagine how your joints, limb position, and muscles might work. By developing a series of highly reliable biomechanical cues, you will be able to master even the most complex of sports by becoming a great motor learner. With no innate skill whatsoever, I have mastered a range of sports, from ski mountaineering racing to kite surfing. Adding these sports is a great intellectual exercise and will add immeasurably to the pleasure in your life.

SUP COACHING

Here are coaches I have used and recommend, should you decide SUP is your sport:

Downwinding

Jeremy Riggs (Maui): I spent seven years training with Jeremy, a Master who really pushes and directs you incredibly well through the water.

Jaecey Suda (Maui): Jaecey has great technical basics and a good eye. He is fantastic at teaching you how to read the water and will take you out on an OC2 (a two-person outrigger canoe) to get a closeup view of the water.

Dave Kalama (Maui): Dave is the original SUP champion and is incredibly helpful on the back end of your stroke.

Jeff Chang (Oahu): There is no better coach at correcting errors and getting you great in the sloppy waters off of Koko Head.

Racing

Larry Cain (Canada): Carolina Cup champion and Toronto Olympics gold and silver medalist, Larry is the master of the classic stroke, and he has superb videos that show these in exquisite detail.

Michael Booth (Australia): The Australian Master was the best in the world in the summer of 2019. He has an incredibly stable and powerful stroke.

Tommy Buday (Burlington, Vermont, and Montreal, Canada): Tommy is an incredibly energetic coach with a dynamic style. He is beloved by our whole club. I spar with Tommy every week and always learn amazing stuff.

April Zilg (Santa Barbara, California): She is the best at beach start lessons. Off like a fighter jet on alert, she is becoming one of the top paddlers.

Connor Baxter (Maui): Connor has the most advanced stroke concept and teaches you a deep blade insertion and powerful back end. I spent a ton of time with Connor.

Travis Grant (Oahu): Travis is the master of the Molokai Channel. He will teach you an incredibly powerful technique.

RESISTANCE TRAINING

Long-time US Ski Team Coach Marty Hall took me aside with a challenge: "How much can you bench?" Marty and I worked together with the US Nordic Team in the late 1970s. I looked at Marty, who appeared incredibly strong and young—early sixties, I guessed. "How old are you?" I asked. "Eighty-one," he answered. I was stunned. A lifelong cross-country ski racer and coach, Marty exuded youth and all the benefits of a huge VO2 max. "Without strength, you got nothing" was his motto. And he's right. I have a close friend I train with in Stowe who is an aerobic superstar, still climbing the Himalayas at age 75. But he has surrendered his muscle mass, and I worry about him. Why? With the loss of strength, he has become frail, and with frailty comes vulnerability to bone fracture and long-term disability.

Aging, even without illness, leads to large decreases in skeletal muscle mass, strength, and function. Here are the frightening numbers associated with this decreased resilience and vulnerability to catastrophe. You'll lose as much as 5 percent of your muscle mass every decade beginning as young as 30 years old, adding up to a 30 percent loss over a lifetime.[45] This increases the risk of having a low-trauma fracture from a fall, such as a broken hip, collarbone, leg, arm, or wrist by 2.3 times, reports the American Society for Bone and Mineral Research.[46] The great news is that you can put that muscle back on, even into your ninth decade. A Medicine & Science in Sports & Exercise article reviewed forty-nine studies of men ages 50–83 who did progressive resistance training; the authors found that study subjects averaged a 2.4-pound increase in lean body mass. A great friend of mine, Bill Evans, undertook a study of 90-year-old volunteers over eight weeks of high-intensity weight training. Volunteers increased strength and functional mobility by an average of 174 percent.[47] The key, Bill said, is high intensity. I see so many people with little five-pound hand weights who are achieving nothing more than toning their muscles.

Ultimately, the number-one, most important exercise as you age is weight training, says Dave Nieman, DrPh, director of the Human Performance Lab at the North Carolina Research Campus. Muscle mass protects you against frailty as you age. Studies show that with training, no age-related muscle loss occurs in the major muscles of the thigh.[48] As a long-distance runner, for example, you may lose a great deal of muscle mass in your eighties, ultimately making you frail—if you don't include weight training.

45 https://www.health.harvard.edu/staying-healthy/preserve-your-muscle-mass
46 https://www.health.harvard.edu/staying-healthy/preserve-your-muscle-mass
47 https://www.researchgate.net/publication/20814302_High-Intensity_Strength_Training_in_Nonage-narians_Effects_on_Skeletal_Muscle
48 https://www.ncbi.nlm.nih.gov/pubmed/?term=Chronic+Exercise+Preserves+Lean+Muscle+Mass+in+-Masters+Athletes

As such, strategies for both prevention and treatment are necessary for the health and well-being of older adults.[49]

The key principle in strength training is to provide a progressive and intense stimulus to the very biggest muscle groups. These are best trained in what are termed compound exercises, which cross multiple joints and target the biggest muscles. Here are the chief advantages:

It builds the most muscles.

It is the safest.

It builds highly functional power and strength.

It builds balance and coordination.

It is the most time efficient.

You don't need a huge range of these exercises. The ones I recommend are below. If you're pressed for time, you can undertake an even shorter list. Ideally, though, you would have ten exercises that you perform two to three times a week.

I'm always stunned at how quickly weight lifting works, and how fast you can lift greater amounts of weight. Over as little as three months as a novice weight lifter, you can achieve a 100 percent improvement in strength. The nervous system adapts very quickly, so that you are recruiting more muscle fibers in a much more coordinated and synchronous manner to improve strength. Older athletes will find that many of their gains are to this neurological adaptation. Over time, your muscle will increase in size as well.

Older athletes will need 25-30 grams of high-quality proteins that include branched chain amino acids immediately after a workout to stimulate the production of new muscle. Younger athletes will need an additional 10 grams. Whey protein is the highest quality and the most easily available source. Older athletes trying to put on muscle need 1–1.3 grams of protein a day per kilogram of body weight. So, a 200-pound man would require as much as 118 grams a day. A 120-pound woman would need to consume 70 grams of protein.

---

49 https://www.ncbi.nlm.nih.gov/pubmed/31343601

Free weights: I admire the discipline of athletes who are able to use free weights, and I would encourage you do to so, if you have the skill and an available spotting partner. However, modern machines take all of the risk out of weight training, allowing you to start with very small loads and working your weight up. For instance, you might not be able to do a single pull-up. However, on a Cybex pull-up machine, you could do dozens and incorporate dips. I'm a huge fan of combining complementary compound exercises. For instance, some machines combine a dip with a pull-up, so you can alternate sets, pull-ups, dips, pull-ups, dips, pull-ups, dips. This is incredibly time efficient.

How many repetitions do you need? Choose a weight that you can only do twelve times before you just can't lift another one. Once you can easily do 8-12 repetitions of your new weight, increase the weight so you again can only do 8-12. Continue this as you progress. Take one day a week for your upper body and another for your legs. If you're in the gym most days for your workout, you may increase this to four days a week, with two each for upper body and two each for legs. If you're adding a third day, you could do lighter weights for up to thirty reps, as coach Tommy Buday recommends for aerobic athletes.

Key compound weight-training exercises: These are exercises that involve multiple joints and muscle groups for the greatest stimulus in building and retaining muscle mass. As an example, a squat involves the quads, hamstrings, and glutes while using the hips, knees, and ankles.[50] You'll train many muscle groups at once and be able to lift more weights than if you perform isolated exercises, such as a biceps curl.

Pull-ups
Tricep dips
Bench press
Leg press
Overhead press
Deadlift

---

50 https://legionathletics.com/compound-exercises/

Cable pulldown

Row

Squat

Shrug

Foam rolling:[51] I've found that with training hard and getting older, the biggest recovery problem becomes muscle soreness, so I've made foam rollers a part of my daily routine. The technical term is Self Myofascial Release. The principle of foam rolling is applying pressure to your muscles with your body weight, then rolling along the length of the muscle. This loosens up the connection between the muscle and the underlying supporting tissue, which is the glue that holds muscle together (also called fascia). I'll complete a workout with tremendous muscle pain and find after just fifteen minutes of foam rolling, 80 percent of the soreness is gone. While deep massage therapy would be ideal, it's impractical on a daily level. If you've never tried this before, just use it on your quadriceps, and you'll find immediate relief, even as you're still rolling. I take a foot-long foam roller in my carry-on bag whenever I travel, so I can foam roll in my hotel room, tent, bunk, or wherever I'm sleeping.

What foam rolling does: Rolling your muscles improves the joint's range of motion. Immediately after rolling my quads, I notice that my knee mobility has improved by 20 percent. After exercise, foam rolling enhances recovery and reduces the onset of muscle soreness.

Conventional size: 6*36

Ideal for travel: 6*18

THE EVIDENCE

A systematic review in the International Journal of Sports Physical Therapy concluded that foam rolling:[52]

---

51 https://www.ncbi.nlm.nih.gov/pmc/articles/PMC4637917/
52 https://www.ncbi.nlm.nih.gov/pmc/articles/PMC4637917/

Increases short-term joint range of motion

Reduces pain

Prevents loss of muscle performance

Three consecutive days of foam rolling was shown to:[53]

Enhance strength and performance

Delay the onset of fatigue

A meta-analysis concludes that foam rolling functions better as a warmup than as a recovery strategy.[54]

Another study demonstrates that form rolling prevents muscular fatigue and generates recovery from muscular fatigue following participation in team sports.

When to foam roll: Coach David Spinney always has his clients always foam roll before stretching. David recommends the rumble roller as the only foam roller that can dig into soft tissue and get directly at the basics efficiently. It's the next best thing to your own massage therapist!

Foam rolling exercise:[55] Here's an example for your all-important quadricep muscles. Begin high up on the muscle, toward the hip. Roll down your quads toward the knee, but don't roll over the joint itself. When you begin, this could really hurt, so you can vary the amount of weight you're pressing down onto the roller with. With time, foam rolling will feel as good as a great massage therapist. Try for twenty full trips down your quad and back up.

MUSCLE ELASTICITY

With increasing age, one of the biggest barriers to performance is the brittleness and stiffness of muscle. Restoring muscle elasticity

53 https://www.ncbi.nlm.nih.gov/pmc/articles/PMC5993692/
54 https://www.ncbi.nlm.nih.gov/pmc/articles/PMC4637917/
55 https://www.ncbi.nlm.nih.gov/pubmed/31024339

and choosing sports that enhance elasticity are key youth-restoring exercises. Cycling is a great example.

Yoga: While plyometrics are a terrific way to build elasticity, these exercises become riskier with aging. And stretching just doesn't go far enough. I much prefer yoga. Here's why. A simple stand-in quad stretch that many runners perform before their workout extends the joint to perhaps 80 percent. Meanwhile, a well-practiced yoga pose could increase that to 120 percent, giving you vastly extended benefits. And I have found it is far more effective. I've learned the full routine of Bikram poses, and I do the ones I need every day. Practitioners developed many poses in India specific to medical conditions. I'd recommend sitting in on a few classes to learn the finer points of technique, so you get the very most out of them.[56]

Standing, deep breathing
Half-moon pose
Hands to feet
Awkward pose
Standing head to knee
Standing bow pose (This tremendously outperforms a traditional
    quad stretch)
Bow pose
Half-tortoise pose
Fixed-form pose

56 https://www.bikramyogaseacliff.com/hotyogasanfrancisco/bikram-hot-yoga-seacliff-postures/

PART II:

FUEL

POLYPHENOLS:

THE FUEL OF YOUTH

"Bob, Bob, you've got to look at this paper! I just emailed it," wrote Dave Nieman, one of the world's preeminent exercise scientists and director of the Human Performance Lab at the North Carolina Research Campus. I clicked the email attachment and began to read it in astonishment. The paper reported a 30 percent decline in all-cause mortality for those who consumed the highest amounts of polyphenols in their diet. To put that into perspective, there is nothing across the entire spectrum of medicine that can compete with that 30 percent decline: no statin, antihypertensive, antibiotic, or operation. The polyphenols in green tea, coffee, fresh fruits, fresh vegetables, olive oil, and red wine serve as incredibly potent anti-inflammatory agents. The beneficial effects derive from reducing inflammation and oxidative stress in the body.[57]

We've seen that inflammation is a major driving force behind many chronic diseases, from heart disease to depression. As an antidote, polyphenols are proving to be the most powerful anti-inflammatory nutrients when it comes to dampening that inflammation and the inflamm-aging from the fight-or-flight switch of our automatic

57 The Journal of Nutritional Epidemiology: High Concentrations of a Urinary Biomarker of Polyphenol Intake Are Associated with Decreased Mortality in Older Adults 1, 2

nervous systems. The polyphenol breakthrough fundamentally recasts nutrition to focus on what we drink as much as what we eat. Building on the core diet of the most successful super-agers, we'll add the beverages and smoothies that deliver the whole spectrum of polyphenols. These beverages add an incredible sensory element—from artisanal coffees to matcha teas to vintage red wines to high arctic blueberry juice. Dave believes the benefit may be even larger, a 30-60 percent decrease in all-cause mortality.

Why polyphenols work: We've learned that mitochondria lie at the heart of youth. The inflammatory processes and inflamm-aging inflict their greatest damage to the mitochondria. The high polyphenol diet is aimed squarely at protecting these factories of youth.[58] Research demonstrates that polyphenols decrease oxidative stress and inflammation within part of the brain called the hypothalamus, which is responsible for the production of new mitochondria. Damage to neurons may play a role in a host of brain diseases, from depression to degenerative neurological illnesses. Polyphenols enhance antioxidant defense systems to stem the degeneration of neurons. Researchers report an inverse association between total polyphenol intake and the risk of overall mortality. This finding was independent of any other nutrients you might be taking or your diet. So, even if your diet isn't fantastic, you'll benefit from a high polyphenol intake.

Best of all, polyphenols signal you that you are succeeding by making you feel better through your improved mood and physical well-being. I fuel myself to feel better and better all day long, following this credo: "Control your mood through your food." I say, "Feel better, be better," through foods that let you know you're succeeding.

Polyphenols in the fit individual: When high-flavonoid intake from fruits and vegetables is bundled with other good lifestyle habits (no smoking, regular physical activity, healthy body weight), the average individual is expected to live six to fifteen years longer than those with none of these good health habits.[59]

---

58 https://www.ncbi.nlm.nih.gov/pubmed/31300352
59 (Am J Public Health. 2011;101:1922–1929; Arch Intern Med. 2009;169:1355-1362; JAMA. 2011;306:62-69; PLoS Med 2012;9(11):e1001335; JAMA. 2012;307:1273-1283).

"By consuming more flavonoids from fruits and vegetables, and adopting good lifestyle habits, individuals have the power to position themselves on a higher survival track." This was observed in research that followed. 4,232 women and men for eleven years.[60]

Polyphenols work even in the sedentary: A new Danish study shows an even more powerful protective effect of polyphenols in smokers, drinkers, and those who are overweight,[61] so the benefits run the spectrum of lifestyles from super fit to not so fit!

THE SPECIFICS

Let's take a more detailed look. A review of thirteen studies with 344,488 subjects concluded that the higher your intake of flavanols, the lower your risk of coronary artery disease. How much? For every 10mg-per-day intake, the risk was reduced by 5 percent. Flavanoids are plant nutrients that give most fruits and vegetables their brilliant colors and work as incredibly powerful antioxidant compounds that have extraordinarily powerful inflammatory effects throughout all the major organs of our bodies. While assembling a variety of fruits and vegetables will go a long way toward this goal, this review adds much greater precision by singling out the six most powerful classes of flavanoids: flavonols, anthocyanidins, proanthocyanidins, flavones, flavanones, and flavan-3-ols. Let's take a look at the best examples of each for your nutritional planning. You'll want one or two from each of these groups every day.

Flavonols:[62]
Here are the most six prominent flavanol groups:

Anthocyanidins: The list shows the most prominent anthocyanidins. Daily blueberry consumption for six weeks increases NK (nat-

---

60 (Int J Cardiology 2013;168:946–952).
61 https://www.nature.com/articles/s41467-019-11622-x
62 https://nutrition.ucdavis.edu/sites/g/files/dgvnsk426/files/content/infosheets/fact-pro-flavonol.pdf

ural killer) cell counts, and acute ingestion "reduces oxidative stress and increases anti-inflammatory cytokines":[63]

Blackberries
Blueberries
Cherries
Cranberries
Eggplant
Grape juice
Plums
Prunes
Raisins
Red apples
Red beans
Red beets
Red cabbage
Red or purple grapes
Red onions
Red pears
Red wines
Strawberries

Proanthocyanidins:[64] Here are the best sources of proanthocyanidins:

Red grapes
Black grapes
Grape seeds
Red wines
Bilberries
Cranberries
Strawberries

---

63 Effect of blueberry ingestion on natural killer cell counts, oxidative stress, and inflammation prior to and after 2.5 h of running; Lisa S. McAnulty, David C. Nieman, Charles L. Dumke, Lesli Shooter, Dru A. Henson, Alan C. Utter, Ginger Milne, and Steven R. McAnulty
64 https://www.urmc.rochester.edu/encyclopedia/content.aspx?contenttypeid=19&contentid=Proanthocyanidins

Blueberries

Red cabbage

Apple peel

Pine bark

Leaves of the bilberry bush

Birch

Ginkgo biloba

Flavones:[65] There are just a few of these. Several supplements also contain flavones but were not included in the studies, since their value is unknown:

Parsley

Celery leaf

Hot peppers

Extract of C. morifolium tablets

Cooked artichoke heads

Flavanones: These citrus fruits are terrific ways to start your day:

Grapefruit juice, white, fresh

Grapefruit, white, raw

Lemon juice, fresh

Lemon, raw

Orange juice, fresh

Orange, raw

Pomelo juice, fresh

Flavan-3-ols: These are easily accessible through apples, teas and wines:

Apples, Red Delicious, raw, with skin

Apricots, raw

65 https://www.livescience.com/52524-flavonoids.html

Chocolate, dark
Tea, black, brewed
Tea, green, brewed
Tea, oolong, brewed
Tea, white, brewed
Wine, red, Shiraz

BEVERAGES

We've seen how beverages may prove to be the best way for you to enjoy a high intake of powerful polyphenols each day and in a highly enjoyable way! Let's have a look:

Coffee

As I wrote in The Coffee Lover's Bible, coffee may be the greatest nutritional miracle in our world today. What other delicious beverage gives you such a bright, consistently optimistic outlook every morning? By drinking the right cup of coffee, you will see a tremendous impact on your overall health, well-being, and longevity. Beyond being the ultimate superfood, coffee is one of the greatest indulgences, a sensory experience that rivals the finest wines. There's simply no other measure you can take to improve your health that requires minimal effort and imparts such amazing rewards. Most telling is an article in The New England Journal of Medicine concluding that women could decrease all-cause mortality by 15 percent with four-five cups of coffee a day, and men could have a 10 percent decrease with five-six cups of coffee a day. If you're part of the 45 percent of the population that processes caffeine slowly and grows jittery with this much caffeine, consider high-quality decafs. The article showed decaf worked as well as caffeinated coffee. High-altitude lighter roasts, such as an Ethiopian Hambela or Kenyan Nyeri are good examples.

Red Wine

Resveratrol is a powerful polyphenol found in red wine with a reputation enhanced by a famous Morley Safer report on 60 Minutes years ago. The story identified resveratrol as the ingredient in red wine that might extend life expectancy. His piece did emphasize that very high concentrations were necessary for the longevity effect, so that a pill might be required instead of drinking several bottles of red wine a day. Laboratory animals protected by resveratrol are drinking up to 1,000 times what humans consume. However, recent observations of the most successful aging populations show consumption of one to two glasses day of a red wine particularly high in polyphenols. Sardinians savor a wine made from homegrown Cannonau grapes, which has as much as three times more polyphenols than the average red wine. Your local wine shop can order this for you. Resveratrol may also boost the absorption of other flavonoids.[66]

RESEARCH

The European Society of Cardiology reported that moderate wine drinking and regular exercise shows protection against heart disease.

The Research Center for the Study of Alzheimer's Disease and Memory Disorders also postulates that resveratrol may prevent the formation of plaques that are linked to Alzheimer's disease.[67]

Alcoholic beverage consumption: If you don't currently drink, I wouldn't advise starting now to enhance your longevity prospects. However, if you do drink regularly, consider red wines that have a very high resveratrol content. There are also high-resveratrol, non-alcoholic red wines to consider. Relative to other polyphenols, resveratrol is not a big player. The most important consideration with alcohol is its affect on sleep. If you are scoring poorly on your sleep

66 https://www.bluezones.com/2017/08/longevity-link-how-and-why-wine-helps-you-live-longer/
67 https://www.ncbi.nlm.nih.gov/pmc/articles/PMC4261550/

measurements, waking up for long periods of time during the night, or waking up groggy, consider drinking less alcohol and drinking it earlier. Do try several nights without alcohol and observe if your sleep scores are substantially improved, using WHOOP, Garmin, or other devices that record and measure REM and deep sleep. If they do improve, you may want to limit or eliminate alcohol consumption. I have tried a non-alcoholic wine. It didn't taste great, and I didn't buy more after we finished that bottle. People often ask me why I don't drink much. Half-kiddingly, I say, "Vanity!" When I first started appearing on the Today show, I noticed bags under my eyes and halting answers. There was a Wall Street Journal article indicating that even one glass of alcohol in the evening ruined productivity the following morning. I stopped drinking, and the clarity of my answers vastly improved! WHOOP also shows that alcohol has the worst effect of all variables on our recovery scores.

Green Tea

Green tea has a special polyphenol called epigallocatechin-3-gallate. High quality matcha green teas may have seven times more of the epicatechins than regular green teas do. A recent National Institutes of Health review concludes that long-term green tea consumption may be beneficial in treating obesity, diabetes, and cardiovascular risk factors.[68]

THE MASTER LIST

Finally, let's look at a master list of polyphenols, ranked from the very most powerful. High-bush blueberries sit on top. I put many of these in my morning smoothie to get a huge polyphenol boost each morning. Although these have the very highest amounts, you do want a variety of polyphenols, as shown in the lists above, even if they don't score at the top of the list, since each has its own specific

---

68 https://www.ncbi.nlm.nih.gov/pmc/articles/PMC2855614/

benefits. It's this variety in healthy populations that carries the day and is associated with decreased all-cause mortality. So, to be super-clear, since it can be confusing, polyphenols are the master category of the healthiest nutrients in fruits, vegetables, red wines, coffees, olive oil, and teas. Flavanols are a subcategory, and each of the six categories carry specific benefits that together drive down the risk of all-cause mortality. So, do add the most powerful to your smoothies, but try to have several servings from each of the flavanol categories too.

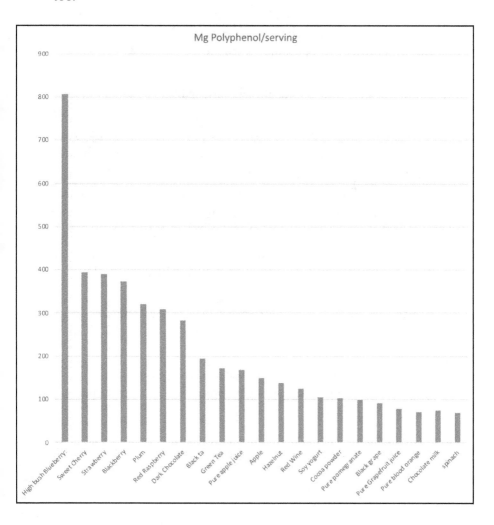

Smoothies

So, you may look forlornly at the list of high-polyphenol foods and sigh, sure, Dr. Bob, that's a really great idea, but how on earth can I consume those during an ordinary day? The answer is simple: smoothies! Why? Because you can pack more nutrition into one morning smoothie than most Americans get in a month. Since these drinks disguise the taste of veggies like kale and collard greens, you can bravely assault a tabletop of amazing fruits and vegetables with nary a fear of choking on veggies that you may hate. Here are the key principles that explain why smoothies work so well in disguising the taste and smell of veggies you may not like:

Freezing: I only shop once a week, buying blueberries, cantaloupe, kale, spinach, collard greens, etc., and I place them in the freezer. Since fresh veggies lose their nutritional value so quickly, freezing stabilizes the nutrient value for the whole week. However, the best part of freezing veggies is that freezing them completely kills the taste. As a small child, I detested most veggies and could barely stomach them. Now I heroically consume a huge amount—because I can't taste a thing. (Of course, if you love them, don't let me stop you from preparing them in any way you wish.) Freezing them also gives your smoothie the consistency and cool temperature of a milkshake.

Fruits: The taste of fresh blueberries, blackberries, and cantaloupe does bleed through to add zest to your smoothie.

Honey: Since you're getting so much amazing nutrition, don't be afraid to add enough honey to make your smoothie better than palatable—in fact, terrific!

Banana: I always add half of a fresh banana to give the smoothie some texture and taste.

Base: I prefer 0 percent (fat-free) Greek yogurt as a base to get much-needed protein. You can also use coconut milk or almond milk. Here's the comparison of protein scores between them. You can see that Greek yogurt leads the pack:

Greek yogurt: 14-16 grams/serving, because the process used to
    make it concentrates the fluids
Almond milk: 4-6 grams
Coconut milk: 2-4 grams

Blenders: Only one blender works for me when it comes to grinding up hard, frozen fruits and vegetables, the Vitamix blender. I have used this brand for decades. When it breaks, customer service is abysmal, but otherwise it's a great and robust product.

I recommend having a large thermos bottle so you can prepare this first thing in the morning, and then carry it with you, sipping on it throughout the entire morning. You could also consider adding another smoothie for dinner to get a double boost of polyphenols and anti-inflammatory fruits and veggies.

Here are some sample smoothies:

My Go-to Smoothie

1 cup water
2–4 tablespoons chia
1/2 cup plain, nonfat Greek yogurt (almond and coconut milk are good substitutes)
1/2 cup frozen blueberries
1/2 cup frozen cantaloupe
1/2 banana
3 cups chopped, stemmed, frozen kale leaves
1/2 cup frozen spinach
1 teaspoon wild honey, or to taste (Make it taste good!)

Combine the water, chia, yogurt, blueberries, cantaloupe, banana, kale, spinach, and honey in a blender. Blend until smooth.

Coco Mango

11⁄2 cups coconut water

1 cup mango, fresh or frozen

1 small banana, fresh or frozen

2 cups firmly packed spinach

3 tablespoons pumpkin seeds

Combine the coconut water, mango, banana, spinach, and pumpkin seeds in a blender. Blend until smooth.

Grapefruit Avocado

1 cup fresh-pressed apple juice

1 cup sections of grapefruit and any extra grapefruit juice

1 cup mint

1⁄2 small avocado

1⁄2 cup cilantro

1⁄2 cup water

Combine the apple juice, grapefruit/any extra grapefruit juice, mint, avocado, cilantro, and water in a blender. Blend until smooth.

Açaí Berry

1 cup açaí juice

1 1⁄4 cups blueberries, fresh or frozen

3⁄4 cup frozen raspberries

1 fresh ripe banana

1⁄4 cup raw cashews

Combine the açaí juice, blueberries, raspberries, banana, and cashews in the blender. Blend until smooth.

Carrot Beet Super Salad

11⁄2 cups fresh pressed carrot juice

1⁄2 cup water

1 cup firmly packed arugula leaves

1⁄2 cup grated raw beets

1⁄2 red apple, core removed and roughly chopped

2 tablespoons raw walnuts

2 tablespoons lemon juice

1 teaspoon flax oil or olive oil

CHRONO-NUTRITION

An important emerging nutritional field is chrono-nutrition, which demonstrates how food and nutrients affect our body clocks and even the clocks of individual genes. Our body's master clock precisely and carefully orchestrates a huge range of hormones and metabolic activities. This is carefully regulated by light and darkness, when and how well we sleep, and when we rise each morning. We feel so terrible after an overnight flight to Europe because our natural rhythms are badly disrupted. However, new research shows that what and when we eat can also enhance these natural, undulating rhythms of body hormones as well as badly disrupt them, causing us to feel tired and even damage the machinery in our bodies that controls our weight and metabolic activities.[69] These circadian clocks are distributed throughout our bodies. While the central clock is governed by light

---

69 PMCID: PMC4118017PMID: Nutrients, Clock Genes, and Chrono-nutrition

and dark, the peripheral clocks throughout our bodies are set by when we eat and when we fast, and they can determine weight gain, and how we use nutrients. For instance, a short night's sleep can increase the amount of the weight gain hormone leptin. A strict eating schedule can improve both how well our clocks work and metabolic problems, like blood sugar regulation and weight gain.

Poor nutrition also lowers your HRV score. Skip breakfast and your HRV drops, a clear sign that you are already stressing your body early in the day. A badly disrupted metabolic clock can lead to overeating, obesity, and increases of blood glucose and fats, also affecting HRV. How do you combat this? Set your biological clocks with the precision of a fine Swiss watch with regular eating times and periods where you restrict all intake, ideally from early evening until breakfast. Eating randomly throughout the day, skipping breakfast, eating high-fat foods, and dining well into the night badly disrupt these rhythms. These habits may leave you lacking energy, sleeping poorly, performing badly, and gaining weight, all while suffering from rises in your blood sugar and cholesterol, putting you at risk of diabetes and heart disease. Worst of all are unpredictable and chaotic eating times. A regular breakfast is a great way to set your body clock for the day and a small, early-evening dinner is much preferable to that late-night pizza, which smashes these precision clocks.

A fantastic review of nutrients and circadian rhythms by Hideaki Oike, Katsutaka Oishi, and Masuko Kobori in the journal Current Nutrition Reports concludes: "The prevalence of metabolic diseases has increased in many countries where circadian behaviors, including mealtimes, can be disrupted and individuals can be deprived of sleep. Time-restricted feeding or a balanced breakfast can powerfully entrain and thus amplify circadian clocks in peripheral tissues, whereas feeding at unusual times or with a high-fat diet attenuates these clocks."

Nutrients also make a huge difference. Polyphenols, fiber, and unsaturated fats improve overall heath while helping to restore the precision of your biological clocks.

So—what a practical application of this incredibly rich and

complex field! I subscribe to the Core Diet for my training and have found it highly effective. Here's a combination:

> Have breakfast at a set time each day.
> Learn to fill up with fruits, veggies, salads, and clean meats during the day.
> Preload with carbs before a workout.
> Reload with a recovery drink.
> Have a light, early dinner.
> Drink a protein shake or take in branched chain amino acids early in the evening.

While training takes discipline, nutritional discipline is much harder, and it is the last frontier for most athletes to conquer. Some never do. Studies of pro athletes[70] conclude they may die earlier than non-athletes. Why? Because they've always had a terrible diet, and when they retire, they continue with the awful diet without retaining the fitness that helped protect them during their professional career.

Here's my typical day, which incorporates the best of chrono-nutrition, and from which I rarely vary:

> 7:00 a.m.: High-polyphenol coffee; Check WHOOP score
> 7:15 a.m.: Protein shake (Klean Isolate)
> 8:00 a.m.: Smoothie (kale blueberry cantaloupe banana)
> 8:30 a.m.: High-polyphenol coffee
> 10:00 a.m.: Low-fat cheese and almonds
> 10:30 a.m.: High-polyphenol coffee
> 12:00 p.m.: Lunch (lean meat and vegetables)
> 12:30 p.m.: Matcha tea
> 2:00 p.m.: Cocoa
> 3:00 p.m.: Low-fat cheese and nuts
> 3:30 p.m.: Large Gatorade
> 3:30–5:00 p.m.: Aerobic workout

---

70 https://www.psychologytoday.com/us/blog/humor-sapiens/201305/comedians-athletes-and-performers-die-younger

5:00 p.m.: Recovery drink
6:30 p.m.: Kale salad and lean grilled chicken
8:00 p.m.: Protein shake

CORE FOODS

My nutritionist has placed me on the Core Diet at the recommenda-tion of my coach. These are the clean foods that should make up the essentials of any good diet. The biggest insight my nutritionist, Ra-chel Gargano, gave me, is that we have to learn to prepare vegetables, salads, nuts, and seeds during the day rather than quick, fast-food fixes. This takes real discipline, but these foods will reward you with a sense of calm, control, and composure. There's lots more on the Core Diet platform (https://www.thecorediet.com):

Fruits: blueberries, raspberries, prunes, strawberries, banana, pineapple, mango, dried figs
Vegetables: broccoli, red bell peppers, asparagus, spinach, sweet potato, butternut squash, purple and green cabbage
Lean proteins (these have the least amount of fat per gram of protein): chicken breast, turkey, fish
Low-fat dairy: Greek yogurt
Nuts
Seeds
Legumes

Packaged foods: Try to avoid these. If you need to buy a bar to eat on the run, the ratio of carbs to protein should be two or less. That is, if there is 10 grams of protein, then no more than 20 grams of carbs or sugars. A good example is the 2.1-ounce GoMacro MacroBar Organic Vegan Protein Cashew Caramel Bar (available on Amazon).

Omega 3 fatty acids: The research runs hot and cold on omega 3 fatty acids. Still I try for a wild-caught Alaskan chinook salmon two to three times a week and a supplement on other days.

Enjoying Carbohydrates

The wrong carbohydrates can wreak havoc on your metabolism by causing large spikes in blood sugar levels. This increases the storage of fat, and you run the risk of diabetes, weight gain, and other illnesses. For those reasons, I eat carbs with a low glucose load during much of the day to settle my blood sugar, give me a sense of calm, and keep my weight stable.

Here are a few carbohydrates that may wreak havoc with your blood sugar:[71]

Doughnuts
French fries
White rice
Instant oatmeal
Pasta
Soda

By contrast, here are carbohydrates that put a much lower load on your system:[72]

Steel-cut oats
Long-grain rice
Whole-grain bread

Carbohydrates are also a terrific performance fuel. Eating these around your training periods allows you to enjoy the high glycemic load of carbohydrates that will improve your performance with no adverse health consequences. Simply put, fuel is speed, and carbs are the raw ingredient that fills our muscle and liver fuel stores, so we can go faster and further while feeling great.

---

71 https://nypost.com/2019/10/26/fdny-medical-lieutenant-charged-with-sexually-abusing-nypd-cop/
72 https://www.health.harvard.edu/healthbeat/a-good-guide-to-good-carbs-the-glycemic-index

PRE-WORKOUT: A CHANCE TO CHEAT!

One of the toughest aspects of maintaining great nutrition habits is staying away from the moderate-to-high glucose load of the carbohydrates we crave. Well, with a great training program, you get a chance to cheat every day while enhancing your performance. One hour prior to your workout, go knock yourself out. Breads, waffles, toast, English muffins, and Fig Newtons are all fair game. If you're not near a kitchen, then gels, power bars, and Clif Bars are all fair game. These faster-burning carbohydrates move through your system quickly, so your digestive system doesn't subtract many resources from your workout efforts. In a previous generation, a steak was a de rigueur pre-game nutritional hallmark. However, protein and fat take huge amounts of resources away from performance during the game, and they are now shunned.

The principal is a simple one. When your body can mainline carbs, do it! I take bike racer Kate Courtney's advice and cook some whole wheat waffles an hour before a big workout.

Water: Trainers advocate .75–1 ounce of water per pound of body weight a day. So, at 200 pounds, I'd be drinking 150 ounces. Many athletes, including New England Patriots quarterback Tom Brady, swear by the high-water-intake strategy. How do you know you have enough? If you watch your stream when you void, a clear stream shows you are fully hydrated. The darker your stream, the less well hydrated you are. Physiologists dispute that we need this much water, so I'll leave it up to your good judgment as to what to drink. The only advice I would leave you with is this: Try to front-load your day with fluid, so that you don't have to get up during the night to relieve yourself, hurting your sleep. With a large smoothie, a protein beverage, and several cups for coffee, I front-load my day.

Competition fueling: The Blackburn Challenge is New England's toughest water race. SUPs, kayaks, surf-skis, dories, and rowing shells line up for staggered starts around Massachusetts's Cape Ann. The current and wind play against you for nearly the entire 19.5 miles. In 2015, the SUP division began with an aggressive start. Half a dozen SUPs sprinted off the start line and into the distance ahead of me. My chance of a win appeared small, and yet I had great confidence in superior distance training and fueling. Strapped to my board were eight Gatorades, with the plan to consume two each hour. Like most SUP athletes, the leaders prided themselves on carrying very little fuel, as little as a liter on their backs. As the ten-mile mark came up approaching a narrow inlet, I reeled in two of the pack. By mile 18.5, I thought I had won but spied one last racer. Even after three hours of paddling hard, I dug in harder and increased my pace, slowly reeling in the last racer, a 25-year-old who usually topped the podium. Twenty minutes later, I finished in first place for SUP. Two attractive women asked me, "Where is David?" "David who?" I queried, half in jest. So how did a 69-year-old beat an incredibly fit 25-year-old? Sure, equipment, training, technique, and experience all played a role. However, proper race-day fueling gave me the much higher fuel stores needed to keep a higher pace right up to the end. In the 32-mile Molokai 2 Oahu Paddleboard World Championships, even after seven hours, I felt just as strong and energetic at the end as the beginning. Properly fueling for training, events, and competitions will add immensely to your enjoyment and success. Let's take a look:

Carbohydrate loading: Just like you'd top off a race car before a big event, you need to top off your fuel stores before a competition, fun ride, or other long-distance event. The more carbohydrates you have stored, the faster you'll go. Remember the motto, "Fuel is speed." Carb loading has been dramatically transformed since it was first introduced in the 1960s. The technique is much less complex, so look closely at the details. As an example, the big carb loading meal is now two nights before the competition, not the night before. Plus, it's not that big!

Here's what I do, based on great advice from my sports nutritionist Rachel Gargano.

Seventy-two hours before the race: Add 100 ounces of sports drink with a good electrolyte mix. Gatorade Endurance is one such beverage.

Two nights before the race: Enjoy a large pasta or rice dinner, but don't overdo it. Aim for about two and a half cups of pasta or rice, with lean protein and veggies.

The day before race day:

Breakfast: Enjoy all the foods you've been avoiding. Now that big pancake breakfast with syrup, home fries, and toast will help you top off your fuel stores. I add three scrambled eggs. You don't want to walk away from the table feeling full. Aim to eat by 8 a.m.

Snack: Four ounces pretzels

Lunch: A six-inch Subway sandwich with no cheese, veggies, or mayo. Add baked chips.

Snack: A bagel with jelly before 3 p.m.

Dinner: Four ounces of baked chicken with 1.5 cups of pasta or rice without sauce. Rachel Gargano advises going to bed hungry. She can prepare your own customized pre-race plan, determined by the length and type of event.

Pre-race fluids

Seventy-two hours before: 100 ounces of fluids a day to be fully hydrated.

The day before the race: Two 24-ounce sports drinks and 50 ounces of water.

The day of the race: One 24-ounce sports drink. Nurse this throughout the morning.

Race day or event fueling: A great race-day nutrition strategy keeps your muscle and liver fuel tanks topped off, prevents bonking after the start (sudden low blood sugar), and keeps your digestive track empty of hard-to digest-proteins and fats. For instance, a stack-and-eggs pre-competition breakfast from the 1950s era would divert sizable resources to digesting all this fat and protein, slowing you down. That's why faster-burning carbohydrates provide an enormous advantage, since they clear your digestive system quickly. Here's my strategy for longer events like Molokai 2 Oahu, Chattajack, the

Carolina Cup Graveyard Challenge, gravel grinders, and 30–50K Nordic races:

Throughout the morning, nurse a 24-ounce sports drink, so you're well hydrated.

Two and a half hours before the event:

First cup of high-polyphenol coffee.

Scrambled eggs (I get hypoglycemic, so eggs help me as they digest more slowly. Skip these if you don't suffer low blood sugar during long events or races.)

Two cups of applesauce (My coach loves this.)

One banana.

Two scoops of branched chain amino acids.

One hour before the event:

One performance power bar.

Ten minutes before start: I drink a large Gatorade, which prevents hypoglycemia. By drinking it this close to the start, your blood sugar won't spike and crash. Practice drinking a performance drink ten minutes before all your hard workouts, so your system becomes accustomed to the ingestion of carbohydrates and water. You may opt for a smaller Gatorade or sports drink, if your system can't handle the larger one, or you have a shorter event. I've never bonked with this strategy.

During the race: Again, fuel is speed. Your goal is to preserve as much of your muscle and liver fuel stores for as long as possible. Your body can absorb up to 90 grams of sugars an hour. My strategy is to train my body to use as much sugar as possible, and it's worked incredibly well. At the end of a seven-and-a-half-hour, grueling paddle across the Molokai Channel on a stand-up board, I had energy to spare in the last one and a half miles against a 30-plus-mph wind. So many of my friends pride themselves on fueling lightly, and then they pay the price in poor performance or by dropping out of events. Here's how many carbs you should try to ingest each hour during a race, dependent on its length:

Four hours: 80 grams
Three hours: 60–70 grams
Two hours or less: 50 grams

I take fuel every twenty minutes to divide up the amount, so that a huge amount isn't ingested all at once, which will slow you down. For Molokai 2 Oahu, I'll just drink a small Gatorade every twenty minutes. This has worked incredibly well for six crossings.

So, how do you get that kind of carbs during an event? For the pace of my events, there is simply no time to stop and eat anything. All of the fuel has to be easily ingested. I focus on three different products. The colder the event and the less you sweat, the less water you may need, and the more you can rely on gels and chews.

During each hour of competition or high-intensity training, try one of these strategies:

One 20-ounce Gatorade (36 grams of carbs every thirty minutes.

or

Two Clif Bloks Energy Chews (24 grams of CHO) every twenty minutes.

(I used these all race season, because I can so quickly stuff two in my mouth, losing only a stroke or two. It's super-efficient; I just toss one between each cheek and let them digest.)

or

One Clif Shot Energy Blok (22–24 grams of CHO) every twenty minutes.

These take longer to open and ingest than the Bloks. You also have to fumble with them; consider starting a tear at the top before the race, so they're ready to go. They're fine for cycling and running, where you have time to open and ingest. You'll have a harder time with SUP, since you are using both hands to paddle, making it difficult to stop, take out a pack, tear it open, and ingest. There is a custom belt where you can put multiple shots on for easy access during an event. I do love these for hikes, where you can get such a quick shot of energy easily.

or

Mix and match: For long events, fluid-based energy can be too cumbersome. As an example, for the 31.5-mile Chattajack SUP race, my board was loaded with 200 ounces of Gatorade. This weighs thirteen pounds. My board actually submerged and became super-tippy with the extra weight, so I looked for alternatives. The gels just took too long to pull out, open up, and squeeze on a paddleboard, where it would cost you four or five strokes at a minimum. Grabbing a Gatorade might cost me fifteen strokes. However, consuming Clif Shot Bloks cut the time required to fuel dramatically. I'd tear the package open and keep it in my pocket.

Here is a sample of mixed fueling for consumption each hour for a longer event:

One 20-ounce Gatorade at twenty minutes (36 grams)
Two Clif Bloks Energy Chews at forty minutes (24 grams)
Two Clif Bloks Energy Chews at sixty minutes (24 grams)
Total for 1 hour: 84 grams

Protein: When you are training hard, this is the nutrient most likely to come up short. I supplement several times a day with a whey protein supplement. The Klean company has terrific supplements; I buy both Klean Isolate and Klean Recovery.

My coach recommends an ounce of protein for every pound of body weight when you are in serious training. This translates into several protein drinks a day to supplement good, clean proteins like turkey, chicken, and fish.

PART III:

FIRE: DO GREAT STUFF

OK!!! The DeLorean has taken you back to the future, and as you look around with your 25-year-old body and your bright optimistic outlook, you say to yourself: "What do I do now that I feel so energetic and full of purpose?" You're no longer staring aging and decline in the face. This raises even larger problems, as articulated by Marc Freedman in his superb May 31, 2015 Wall Street Journal piece:

"In the early decades of the 21st century, we are pushing, rapidly, to extend our lives. But we're paying scant attention to how we should make the most of that additional time." Where are the innovations designed to make these bonus decades actually worth living? Aside from the mind-boggling prospect of saving for fifty- or seventy-five-year retirements, how do we make these new chapters both fulfilling for individuals and sustainable for society?"

The answer? Do great stuff! Many of us just don't think of undertaking great or even heroic activities. I've experienced the most spectacular life working with some of the most heroic people on Earth in amazing humanitarian organizations, from Save the Children and the UN High Commissioner for Refugees to Doctors Without Borders. I've also been embedded with US forces in Iraq, Afghanistan, Somalia, Kenya, and the Arabian Gulf for the War on Terror. Below you'll find some examples that have inspired my own life. When you think bigger than yourself, the rewards are multiplied enormously. If you're nervous or anxious about your future, just say to yourself, "Be brave. Be bold." Having a purpose for living lies at the heart of successful aging.

NEVER THINK YOU'RE TOO INSIGNIFICANT
TO MAKE A DIFFERENCE

Many of us think we are just too insignificant to make a difference; that only huge organizations and governments have that capacity. The late Marla Ruzicka taught me how wrong I was. She approached me one morning at the Al-Hamra Hotel in Baghdad in 2003 with a big smile. "We're going to save a life today," she said. Marla was referring to a 4-year-old girl who had burns over 50 percent of her body. She pointed to a Times of London account predicting she would expire that day without advanced burn care. I looked at Marla incredulously, as if to say, "How can the two of us do anything to change that?" Intrigued but doubtful, even cynical, I jumped into a cab and headed to a Baghdad hospital with Marla. In a room that looked like a 13th century dungeon was a poor little girl under a large metal cage with her burns exposed. Marla turned to me and said, "Get me a helicopter." At a loss for words, I walked out of the ward and onto the street outside the hospital gates, where a US Army ammunition carrier was parked. I approached the private standing at the rear door of the vehicle.

"May I have a helicopter for a badly burned young girl?"

"Sure thing, I'll get right on it."

Incredulous and dumfounded, I looked up in the sky fifteen minutes later and saw a Black Hawk Medevac helicopter shadowed by an Apache Gunship attack helicopter, both taking small arms fire. Marla and I scrambled to prepare the girl and two other burn victims, then struggled through the massive traffic jam outside the hospital to the Black Hawk, which had landed in a nearby field. As the helicopter lifted off, the mother of the most severely burned girl pulled at my shirt, crying and begging to go on the helicopter with her daughter. Sadly, there was no room. A week later, I visited the US Army's 28th Combat Support Hospital. The little girl had survived and was thriving. With a big smile on her face, she was surrounded by a large US Army medical team. Several had offered to adopt her. Marla taught me an amazing lesson: Never think you're too insignificant or the task too large to make a heroic effort. Marla went on to found Campaign for Innocent Victims in Conflict (CIVIC, now the Center for Innocent Victims in Conflict), which continues to work on behalf of civilians in today's combat zones, like Syria, where civilian injuries, deaths, and displacements are an everyday occurrence. Tragically, Marla's car was hit by a suicide bomber on the road to the Baghdad airport two years later. Her last words were: "I'm alive, I'm alive." She remained optimistic to her last breath and was an eternal inspiration to those who knew her or were touched by her actions.

BE A HERO

During the famine in Somalia in the early Nineties, Baidoa was "The City of Death," where thousands of young children perished every week. As the staff of the International Medical Corps (IMC) lunched in their secure compound, rocket-propelled grenades detonated in the marketplace. Hearing the explosions, we scrambled to the IMC emergency room. Medical volunteers dragged fifty-four badly injured women and children out of makeshift ambulances and onto beds, stretchers, and the bare floor. Several died before we could help. An EMT opened the belly of a woman and began stitching her lacerated bowel back together. One of the remaining patients was 4-year-old Aisha, who was cold, pale, sweaty, and breathing rapidly. Her pulse was fast and her respirations shallow. Aisha had only hours to live without a blood transfusion. The clinic had no blood bank, but that didn't stop Mickey Richer, a mild-mannered 54-year-old pediatrician from Denver. Angry, Mickey said, "I'm not going to stand by and let another little girl die." Mickey rolled up the sleeve on her left arm and called for Dracula, the nickname given to the clinic's technician. Dracula inserted an IV into Mickey's arm, withdrew a pint of (universal donor) Type O Rh Positive blood, and transfused the young girl. Aisha survived. I asked Mickey how often she had transfused her own blood into her patients. "Maybe fifty times," she said. When you next think of heroism, think of Mickey, who risked her life in a lawless land ruled by warlords to save the lives of others. Mickey led by personal example, donating her own blood. We may not work in a conflict zone, but we have a chance every day to be a hero to others, whether donating a pint of blood or helping a neighbor in trouble.

THINK BIG

Galapagos: Life aboard a Scripps Institute of Oceanography research vessel was pretty routine and dull. The crew was exploring the ocean floor far out in the Pacific Ocean, searching for specialized mineral formations. The boredom lifted when our vessel received a distress call from a super freighter. The vessel's 38-year-old third mate appeared to be suffering a heart attack. Concerned, our captain agreed to rendezvous with the freighter. There was a total eclipse on the same day that we made our way at full speed to the ship. In nearly gale-force winds, I was lowered into a small motorboat and driven to the giant ship. A rope ladder was placed over the side. As the small boat went up and down in large swells, roughly twenty feet at each pass, I waited for my chance, then leapt for the ladder. The crew escorted me to the third mate's room. He had indeed had a severe heart attack and would not survive without help. I volunteered to stay on the freighter. We fashioned an IV line, and I made up an antiarrhythmic formula that we hoped might steady his highly irregular and alarming heart rhythm. Without an EKG monitor, we established a 24-hour watch, where crew members held two fingers loosely over an artery in his wrist to observe if his pulse was still irregular. Once he was stabilized, I climbed to the bridge and asked the captain where we could offload the patient. The captain suggested sailing all the way around Cape Horn and then dropping him off in Brazil. I insisted the ship's officer would not survive that long, which turned out to be accurate. We poured over the charts and found that the remote Galapagos Islands were closest. The captain objected, but I reiterated that he just wouldn't live to see Brazil. Reluctantly, the captain agreed. Now to figure out how to get him from the remote Galapagos to a major cardiac center. I started calling on the ship's radio and was able to talk with the US Air Force personnel at Travis Air Force Base in California. A USAF crew was training in a Lockheed C-130 Hercules transport. The officer in charge volunteered to pick us up on Baltra Island at 6 a.m. two days hence. We re-doubled our efforts to keep the officer safe and comfortable. At dawn that day, a small Ecuadorian Navy vessel rendezvoused with our vessel. I supervised lowering the patient into the Navy boat and then sailed to Baltra Island. As we neared shore, the C-130 flew closely overhead in what was an incredibly dramatic and emotional moment. On shore at the aircraft, we were all searched for weapons and explosives. None here! Medics tended him for the flight to a USAF base in Panama. We flew at low altitude so that he had the maximum amount of oxygen. At the air base, he was transferred to an ambulance and then to a large hospital with a cardiac intensive care unit. As soon as the patient entered the hospital, he suffered a cardiac arrest but was soon revived. Literally two minutes later and it would have been too late. Our timing was perfect. I thought back on how ridiculous the whole adventure seemed. How could a 26-year-old doctor commandeer a giant super freighter and convince the USAF to fly a rescue mission? This gave me great confidence going forward that anything was possible if the objective were noble.

BE POSITIVE IN ADVERSITY

"Hey, you were great on Don Imus this morning," a cheerful Marine Corps officer shouted out at me over the sound of a Boeing CH-46 Sea Knight Marine Corps helicopter with its rotors still spinning as it sat on a berm, with a 7th Marine Regiment combat team in Southern Iraq several days into the US invasion. I was embedded with HMM-365, the Blue Knights, a medium-lift USMC helo company. The Pentagon news summary, called the Early Bird, had an account of the Imus exchange, which the officer had read.

Don began: "Understand the Marines are having a tough time, and that it could be six months until they arrived in Bagdad."

"Who said that?" I asked.

"Oh, you know, the NY Times, CNN, BBC."

"Oh, those guys? Imus, they're around seventy miles behind us with the supply guys. The tennis netting might take six months to reach Baghdad, but I'm confident these Marines will be in Baghdad within the week."

I looked down at the rank on the Marine officer's uniform. There was a star! A general!

"Hey, Bob. It's Kelly. Johnny Kelly. I'm the assistant division commander."

As a highly competitive journalist, I sensed an opportunity. General Kelly asked me what I wanted, and I told him.

"I want to be at the pointy edge of the spear, that is, the lead combat regiment. I want to go with you. I'm betting on the Marines being the first into Baghdad." Soon I was standing with Cowboy John Mayer, the lieutenant colonel who commanded the 1st Marine Regiment combat team. "Make me famous," he said. The next day, he was.

Boom!!! Boom!!! Boom!!!

I stood next to a USMC Humvee with Gunnery Sergeant Tom Parks outside of the town of Al-Kūt, a must-take city for any would-be conqueror of Baghdad. Gunfire erupted all around us. Some of it was outgoing suppressive fire from our roof-mounted 50-caliber machine gun. The rest of it was incoming from fedayeen elements. Our embedded reporter rules were simple: No live broadcasts during ongoing operations that might give away our position to the enemy, and no reporting of strategic or tactical plans. I approached the colonel and said, "Look, I'm no military genius, but judging by the incoming fire, I'd say they know where we are. May we go live?"

"Knock yourself out," was the response. We spun up our live camera.

Alex Witt, the anchor in New York, was astonished by the amount of gunfire and cautioned me.

"Shouldn't you duck?"

"Not sure it's a Marine Corps term, but I will check."

I turned to Tom Parks and asked, "Tom, should we duck?"

"Not much of any place to duck, Bob. You have heavy machine

gun fire coming in from the West, Northwest, North, Northeast, and East," Tom explained.

Some of that fire was directed at Tom by a fedayee. He picked up his M16 rifle with iron sights and shot him. Then the fedayee's hostage, a 14-year-old girl, ran out into the battle space in front of us, carrying a baby. The Marines shouted, "Get back," not knowing if she wore a suicide vest. Captivated by the look of sheer horror on her face, I ran out, grabbed her, and put her down in a ditch to prevent her getting shot. Then I said to myself, "Bob. What have you done now? You're stuck in the middle of a ferocious firefight with a girl and a baby."

A few minutes later the gunfire subsided, and the Marine Colonel yelled at me: "Hey Bob. Want to bring your guests in for lunch?"

I grabbed the baby and took the girl by the hand, leading them into the center of the Marine position. I offered a Meal, Ready-to-Eat (MRE) to her. She selected the chicken, which I began to prepare as fire was concentrated on the area around us by the fedayeen. Two Bell AH-1 Cobra helicopters spun up and concentrated TOW missile fire on the nearby fedayeen position. I grabbed the baby and ran with the girl to three M1A1 Marine Corps tanks, which had just arrived, and took cover behind them. I then raised my microphone, went up to the colonel, and asked him what he thought about the raging battle surrounding him.

"Colonel, you have heavy incoming machine gun fire, your Humvee was almost hit, an RPG landed just yards away. What do you have to say?"

He stood up ramrod straight and stared into the TV camera. "It's a great day to be a US Marine." Lesson learned! Even in the most adverse conditions, never pass up the chance to be an inspiration and to stay positive.

SEIZE THE DAY

After the fall of Baghdad in April 2003, I remained in Iraq reporting for MSNBC as chief foreign correspondent and also as a humanitarian aid worker assessing the most pressing needs. I'd report my findings to the Combined Joint Task Force 7 and Save the Children, where I served as a board member. In the first few days, I visited every hospital in the city, finding dozens of children badly injured during the invasion. Unable to get specialized care for them in Baghdad, I asked for a plane to transport them out of the country for care. The allies had no planes to spare, so I called in a favor from Prince Bandar bin Sultan Al Saud, Saudi Arabia's ambassador to the US. The prince sent a Saudi Arabian National Guard plane to Baghdad. I ran around the city, putting kids in ambulances and taxis to take them to the awaiting plane. The last stop was the Baghdad's Alwaiya Children's Hospital, where dozens of children had acute leukemia. The wards were a horror show, with children all sandwiched together in one large room, each infected and infecting those around them. Because equipment used to treat these children was "dual use" under international sanctions, these children were left without adequate diagnosis or treatment and most would die. I reported this on the air one evening for MSNBC. Shortly afterward, I got a call from Paul Newman, whose international board I served on.

Paul said, "Bob, get those kids out of Baghdad, every one of them. I don't care how much it costs."

The next morning a young mother approached me, cradling her 1-year-old baby Miet in one arm and holding up a brain scan with the other. I looked at the scan and told her Miet had no chance to survive in Baghdad. Did she want to take a chance and go to Amman, Jordan, which had a top-rated children's cancer center? Yes, she said.

This was an opportunity to find a route out for Paul's mission. The following day at 6 a.m., Miet and her mother arrived in an impossibly small compact car, then transferred their belongings to our Suburban. We drove through Ramadi and Fallujah, and on to the border.

The crossing guard looked at the baby and said, "What child gets to cross an international border without a passport? Go back." A Norwegian journalist observed the upsetting interactions, grabbed his satellite phone, and called the director of the King Hussein Cancer Center, Samir Khleif, then passed the phone to me.

"I will immediately accept the care of your child, just bring her to me," Samir said.

"I can't."

"Why not?"

"The border guard won't let us cross."

"That's not a problem."

"Not a problem?"

"No. I'll call the palace."

Of course, I thought. Obviously, just call the King!

Samir reached Prince Al-Waleed bin Talal, a cancer survivor, who called the border guard.

The guard appeared, quivering and sweaty.

"Go. Take your baby."

I walked through a crowd of hundreds of Sunni and Shia Muslims, Chaldeans Catholics, and Kurds, all putting their blessings on the child. In the early evening, we arrived at the hospital. The whole staff had stayed behind for Miet and presented her with a big Mickey Mouse balloon, then inserted an IV.

Samir gave me a stern look and said, "Come to my office." He closed the door and said, "I did you a favor. Now you do me a favor. Get the rest of these kids out of Baghdad and to us here in the Amman."

I quickly organized a team. Air Serv International would fly the children out of Baghdad. IOM, the International Organization for Migration, would help with visas and passports. IMC, the International Medical Corps, would help care for family members left behind. The (US) National Cancer Institute would supply doctors, nurses, training, and medication. In the end, we brought 3,000 children into Amman. The idea was simple. Bone marrow transplants were an unaffordable $500,000 in the US but only $50,000 in Amman. Queen Rania of Jordan and Paul Newman each donated $600,000. The operation was kept quiet for fear of tipping off terrorist elements, who might target the children or NGOs.

Lesson learned: When you see a problem, no matter how big, seize the opportunity to help. You'll have lots of company.

NEVER GIVE UP HOPE

During the Rwandan genocide, more than a million refugees entered Zaire (now the Democratic Republic of the Congo), crossing the Rwandan border at Gisenyi. Unfortunately, there was a cholera carrier who lived on Lake Kivu. As refugees passed the lake, they drank and took additional water supplies with them. Soon thousands were infected with cholera. As the refugees made their way up the road by the base of the active volcano Nyiragongo, tens of thousands fell ill. My CBS camera crew and I walked among the many who lay dead by the side of the road. Among them there was a little boy who had apparently expired. As the cameraman photographed a picture of him from a respectful distance, the audio engineer proclaimed, "He's alive!" I put a small amount of water in a bottle cap and put it beside the little boy's mouth. He sipped it. He was alive! I picked him up, and we took him to the Doctors Without Borders (MSF) camp at Kabumba. MSF had predicted there would be a large-scale cholera epidemic here two years before and had stockpiled supplies, but when we reached the camp, they said they were stretched too thin and did not have the personnel to treat our little boy, whom we had nicknamed Joe.

"I'm a doctor; do you mind if I treat him?" I asked.

"Go ahead!" an administrator said.

I prepared oral rehydration solution (ORS) with water. This life-saving drink was used throughout the third world to treat diarrhea. Several months before, the head of UNICEF, Joe Grant, invited Dan Rather and me to lunch, asking us to do a story on ORS. We said that a story on its own wouldn't make sense, but that there would be a big crisis in which ORS would be a large part of the solution, which we would report. Who could have guessed that just a few months later the biggest refugee exodus in history would occur! However, we had an unwritten rule that when we were caring for patients, we would not report the story, so that the care of the individual was our first—and only—priority, and that every decision was in the best interest of the patient, not the story. Within hours, the little boy was so much better that he began to kick his legs at us. MSF staff said there was no room for him to stay. I picked him and brought him to our truck. He had what is termed dry cholera. That is, he was so dehydrated he could not defecate. However, as I picked him up, loose diarrhea oozed all over his legs and clothing. We transported him to the French Opération Turquoise headquarters at the Goma International Airport. Our team asked an angelic-appearing young nurse if she would care for little Joe.

She said. "Of course, we will care for your little boy."

We were all in tears. Joe disappeared into the mists of history. (Sadly, when children were reunited with their parents two years later, many parents no longer recognized their own children.)

Several days afterward, I started to feel badly ... really badly. I went to the airport and paid $250 for a Ukrainian transport plane to fly me to Nairobi. The plane sat on the runway most of the night, blocked by a USAF C-5B. I spent much of the evening chatting with MSF founder Bernard Kouchner. At dawn, the plane departed for Nairobi. On arrival, I was so sick I could only lie on the hotel room floor, unable to lift my head, drinking Fanta orange soda. I had the classic rice-water diarrhea of cholera. After a day, I summoned enough energy to take a taxi to the Nairobi hospital, where I requested a box of ORS, the same formulation I had given to little Joe.

The physician said, "Let us examine you."

After recording my blood pressure while I was in a recumbent and sitting position, he said, "Unless we admit you, you won't be with us tomorrow morning."

With that inspiring message, he admitted me to a ward in the Nairobi hospital. Lying on a damp mattress and hearing mosquitos buzzing around my head, I asked the nurse what conditions the other patients in the room were suffering from. "Malaria," she said.

I then said, "Well, I have a private room, and I'll be going there soon."

She protested, saying there were no private rooms. I insisted that there were. Lucy Fox, our fixer from CBS News, purchased a box of IV fluids, and the two of us went to the Norfolk Hotel. I hid my two IVS under my double-breasted blue blazer and checked into the hotel. I took down the pictures in my room and used the hooks for the IV bottles. After several days in my private room, I was well enough to travel. I could only think how much more miserable the poor victims of cholera were out in the open air around Goma. As a UNHCR and Save the Children board member, I called on those organizations to re-double their efforts to save these poor souls. As I thought back to our poor little Joe, the words of Mother Teresa rang in my head:

"We cannot all do great things. But we can do small things with great love."

SELFLESS BRAVERY

After the first Gulf War, Saddam Hussein turned his vengeance on the Shia in the south and the Kurds in the north. Soon he had driven tens of thousands of Kurdish families north from their homes into the mountains that formed the border with Turkey. Soon hundreds of small children were dying in the bitter cold, snowy nights high up in the mountains. Sensing a vitally important story, I contacted Scott Air Force Base and asked for transportation on a USAF plane. Our favorite public affairs officer quickly lined up the trip, and we were on our way in the spacious compartment behind the cockpit of the US-AF's largest transport plane, the C-5B. We overnighted at Ramstein Air Base in Germany. This is a fascinating facility, where air force crews from around the world land, rest, eat, and depart for exotic locations. The following afternoon, we landed in Turkey and drove to the regional city of Diyarbakır. Reminiscent of a 19th-century Ottoman city, men sat drinking their Turkish coffee and smoking from long-stemmed pipes. Each day my producer, Tracy Chutorian, and I would drive sixteen hours round trip across the Iraq border to these camps. One story demonstrated how small sewage streams exiting from the tents in the camp drained into larger streams that served as the main source of drinking water. (Our audience observed the cycle of illness and death that afflicted so much of the third world, with diarrhea accounting for the second-largest number of deaths in children worldwide, killing nearly a million children a year.)[73] Once again, Doctors Without Borders was in force in these camps. Many US physicians volunteer for this amazing organization, but this operation was led by the Dutch MSF. Their physicians quickly brought in clean water, stopped children from drinking dirty water, and rerouted the drainage system in the camps. The death rate plummeted. What a joy to see so much good done in such a short period of time. The one episode that still sticks out in my mind is when a Dutch physician tried to pass the line of heavily armed Turkish soldiers to enter the camps.

The Turks said, "You may not pass, or we'll have to shoot you."

The resolute physician said, "You have your job to do and I have mine. I am saving children."

With that he walked through the line of soldiers, rifles aimed at him. No one fired a bullet. They let him pass under the watchful eye of our CBS cameras.

Although these tragedies would appear to be incredibly depressing to observe, the efforts of humanitarian aid officers like this physician inspired all of us who saw this that day. The selfless bravery of this young Dutch physician will stay with me forever.

The one regret that many people have as they face death is not having been true to themselves and their principles. Think how many times we have compromised ourselves or our values with far less risk than death involved. This Dutch physician teaches us all that there are values worth upholding, even in the face of death.

KEEP A SENSE OF HUMOR IN ADVERSITY; IT JUST MIGHT SAVE YOUR LIFE

Somalia suffered a horrific famine in 1991. As an advisory member of the US Committee for Refugees and Immigrants, I had watched our

73 https://borgenproject.org/main-causes-child-mortality-developing-countries/

director, Roger Winter, campaign for several years against the atrocities committed by Somalian President Mohamed Siad Barre, but to no avail. Despite all the warnings, Somalia collapsed into a chaos from which it has yet to recover. I explained to CBS, where I worked as a medical correspondent, that this was a story we needed to cover. CBS Foreign Editor, Allen Alter said there was a new technology, never tried before in Africa, and CBS would like me to go and cover the story. This was a portable satellite dish that allowed us to cover stories from the most remote, dangerous, and desolate parts of the planet. Somalia would prove to be the ultimate test. Our plane made an unscheduled stop in Cyprus to pick up the gear and then landed us in Mogadishu, where we picked up a small army to defend our crew in a state that existed in true anarchy. Each day we drove out of the city, filmed a story, and returned. One day our target was the village of Bur Akaba, which had been especially hard hit. Enroute, we stopped off at a small village where there was a camp run by an Irish charity. Toward the end of our shoot, all the children lined up.

I shouted to them: "Who feeds you?"

In a scene that would bring tears to the eyes of all but the most hardened cynic, they shouted back, "Ireland feeds us!"

Indeed, it did. Ireland had an outsized pretense throughout the most desperate countries and performed remarkable services that saved many children. In the Bur Akaba we set up a live shot. This was a remarkable scene, since for the first time our viewers would be inescapably linked to the death and destruction in Africa as they ate their breakfast. As the show went live, I sat with a young mother and her two children. She had already lost two children and was deeply fearful of losing the others. I walked over to bags of grain, donated by the World Food Programme or the Lutheran Church.

When I attempted to take a bag back to the mother, warlords pointed their guns at me and said, "No!"

What a powerful demonstration to our audience of the selfishness of warlords that prevented these children from surviving.

Years later, in another remote village years suffering from a cholera epidemic, we watched helplessly as children expired. Water pumps had been donated, and these children could have been saved. When warlords visited our camp to see what else they could steal, one brave World Vision International leader stood up and said, "These children would not be dying if you had not stolen the water pumps." The selfishness of these warlords and so many militias throughout war-torn Africa always struck me as among the most selfish and heartless people on Earth.

As the satellite technicians finished packing up the $1.5 million worth of gear, thugs from the local warlord's gang swarmed around the gear, intent on stealing it. My producer, Joe Halderman, and I thought quickly. We grabbed a book of Elvis Presley songs and began singing "I'll have a blue Christmas without you." Hundreds of children gathered, laughed, and tried to sing. Humiliated, the gunmen left.

On the four-hour drive back to Mogadishu, I tried to fashion a script on my laptop computer, but our drivers and guards started yelling and screaming at each other, making the task difficult. By mid-morning, khat was available throughout Somalia. Locals stuffed their cheeks full of the leaves of this mild hallucinogenic drug and were transformed from docile to inane. By early afternoon, a hefty dose of khat lit up driver and guards. I raised my voice and asked them if they could settle down so I could write my script. We were under tight time pressure to have a script written and recorded for the CBS Evening News.

My producer responded, "Hey, Bob. They're on drugs and have guns. They'll do as they please!"

Lesson learned: Every day was like a scene from Monty Python. A sense of humor kept you alive. Humor is one of the most important traits we often lose as we age. A child laughs hundreds of times a day. As adults, we guard against laughter and humor, wanting to appear serious and professional. But laughter is the best medicine. Laughter triggers feel-good endorphins and improves our brain chemistry.[74] Laughter is good for the heart and has an effect similar to antidepressants by releasing serotonin. While remaining respectful, we found

---

74 https://www.forbes.com/sites/daviddisalvo/2017/06/05/six-science-based-reasons-why-laughter-is-the-best-medicine/#22dcbdbe7f04

that laughter made many life-or-death situations better, and in this case, it may have even saved our lives. We laugh less as we age—when we should laugh more. Having a light-hearted attitude helps us get though life's travails tremendously.

BE BRAVE, BE FEARLESS

Roger Winter, Austin Hearst, and a team from the US Committee for Refugees and Immigrants sat around the campfire in southern Sudan with the late legendary rebel commander John Garang. I'd known Dr. John for decades, and he was considered one of the best of a new generation of African leaders. He had just won a major battle in which roughly 1,700 Sudanese Army troops had been killed and 1,800 captured. We visited the POW camp and saw many soldiers were children, some just 12 years old. We considered that the government wanted to retaliate against the southern rebel army for their defeat at their hands. Then word came in late one evening that the Sudanese Air Force might try to bomb us the next morning. Austin and I tried to decide between driving sixteen hours to Uganda or risking a flight on the relief plane the following day. The next day dawned peacefully in this small, iconic village. Thinking there was no danger, we packed up and headed to the airport. Then chaos erupted. We could hear nearby explosions and saw an Antonov aircraft overhead. These Ukrainian transport planes served as makeshift bombers; crew members rolled bombs fashioned from oil drums out the back. Our single-engine Cessna 208 Caravan relief plane landed. Pilots offloaded critically needed medications. Then, amongst the explosions, we entered the aircraft, which quickly took off.

Dmisi, our ex-Ethiopian Air Force MiG pilot, flew the plane south toward Lokichogio, the Kenyan airport used to resupply bases in southern Sudan. Soon we relaxed, apparently out of danger. Then voices were heard on the radio "MiG zero one, MiG zero two, target 178 closing." These fighters from the local air base in Juba were apparently closing in on us. I asked the pilot what we should do. He said the MiGs were very poor when maneuvering at slow speeds, so we did a series of tight circles at 60 degrees bank, seeking cover in large cumulous clouds. This was a seminal moment. I asked myself, how should I feel? We're about to get shot down by MiGs. Should I be scared, frantic, afraid, panicked? I reassured myself that if we got hit, we'd never know it. It was then I discovered that fear was a choice. I chose not to be afraid then or ever again. Dmisi flew out of the clouds, the MiGs vanished, and we landed safely in Lokichogio.

Later in the year, Save the Children CEO Charlie MacCormack, Austin Hearst, and I travelled to the Nuba Mountains to observe Save the Children's relief activities in this key front-line area in the battle between northern and southern Sudan. The jovial local governor welcomed us.

During conversation that evening at dinner, I casually queried, "What was your last job?"

He said, "I ran the air force base in Juba."

I said, "You know, your MiGs targeted a plane earlier this year."

He said, "Yes, I know, this was a rebel aircraft, and we tried our best to shoot him down."

I hesitated, then said, "That was our aircraft. Austin and I were in it."

Without missing a beat, he said, "Oh, we are so glad we missed. Welcome to Sudan. You are our honored guests."

Lesson learned. FDR was right There's nothing to fear but fear itself!

Dateline: Sadr City, Iraq
Embedded: The I Marine Expeditionary Force (I MEF)

Before the Second Persian Gulf War, the NBC news foreign desk sat me down and read me the riot act.

"Look, Bob, you are the most dangerous correspondent we have. I don't want you to take any risks without checking with me first."

"Risks ... like going to a live war?" I thought as I was being dispatched to join the US Marine Corps I Marine Expeditionary Force in Kuwait, where it was preparing for invading Iraq.

That same voice came on the satellite phone many months later, as a 1st Marine Regiment team sat outside of Bagdad.

"Look, Bob, the Iraqis are pulling down the statue of Saddam Hussein in Firdos Square. There are no embedded reporters in downtown Baghdad. You're closest. Could you make your way to Firdos Square?"

I couldn't stop myself from saying, "But it's dangerous." Then I agreed.

Tom Parks, the RCT-1 gunnery sergeant, arranged to drive me to downtown Baghdad from Sadr City. Barbed wire and checkpoints were at nearly every street corner. Tom put a 9mm pistol next to me just in case.

The Marine Humvee got about halfway from the Sadr City cigarette factory to Firdos Square when the Marine driver said, "Sorry, you'll have to get out, it's too dangerous."

So, I stood out in the street with a full US Marine Corps flight suit on, $60 in my pocket, a passport, and nothing else. After years of living in New York City, I had learned to be resourceful. I stuck my hand up and yelled, "Taxi!"

Soon a tiny, badly dented, yellow Iraqi cab picked me up and drove me to the center of the action. About 100 yards from the Palestine Hotel on Firdos Square, the driver dropped me off. I dashed toward the finish line in the journalist Olympic Games to be the first embedded reporter to make it to downtown Baghdad and witness Saddam's teetering statue. Navy medics stopped me, asking for help with two young boys who had been shot in the crossfire. After assisting and getting them into ambulances, I continued to the NBC broadcast platform in the Palestine. NBC's Iraqi crews maintained a live camera vigil for the entire war. The crew and I hugged each other, knowing we were now safe. Soon Tom Brokaw and Katie Couric were on the line. They asked me how relieved I was that the war was finally over. "Over?" I asked in a puzzled voice. "Do you know the history of this country? This isn't the end. This is the beginning." Still it was a great feeling competing against the best journalists in the world and beating them to the fall of Baghdad!

PART IV:

THINK BIG TO FEEL GREAT

The former CEO of a Fortune 500 company approached me in the Yale Club main lounge.

"What are you doing professionally?" he asked.

I named a series of humanitarian, health technology, writing, and television projects.

Thoughtfully, he responded, "Bob, do you know what you're actually doing?"

"No," I answered.

"You are leading the portfolio lifestyle."

He explained that many successful individuals increased their impact by embarking on a complementary series of projects folded into a portfolio of work instead of having a single job. I loved the many wonderful projects I'd undertaken, from the excitement of researching them to the sense of fulfillment and pride in the final product. I also had a diverse learning portfolio from languages and music composition to deep learning. I always wondered why I was drawn to multiple work projects and a broad learning portfolio. Harvard Psychiatrist Moshe Bar constructed the most fabulous theory, which I adhere to. Moshe[75] hypothesized that broad associative thinking promotes a positive mood. From an evolutionary viewpoint, this makes sense, since broad associative thinking stimulated us to invent and pioneer. This thinking brought us from the discovery of fire and construction of stone wheels to iPhones and artificial intelligence. Our brains are rewarded for this broad activity and stimulation by improving our mood and lending us even more mental energy to take on greater challenges. The associative piece is key, since your brain works hard to make many new connections. For instance, in learning to code a computer program or speak a

75 https://www.ncbi.nlm.nih.gov/pmc/articles/PMC2767460/

language, your brain creates millions of new connections. I lead my life with a portfolio of creative projects and a constant portfolio of learning among diverse topics, from language to machine learning. With the tremendous physical energy that you'll enjoy from dynamic training, you'll have an unbridled enthusiasm to be intellectually active. Create for yourself a portfolio of learning that follows your passions and you'll find your mood will soar.

THE GIG ECONOMY

With today's fast-paced changes in every industry and the advent of the gig economy, keeping ahead of the educational curve is vital to survival and success. I recommend always having a portfolio of learning, where you tackle big, challenging, new subjects. You'll recall the theory that it just takes 10,000 hours to become a world-class expert at anything. That's ten years of twenty hours a week or five years of forty hours a week. Clearly you can become extremely good without being a world-class expert in less time. We've grown up with the idea of educating once and then stretching what you have learned out for a long career. The new thinking is that we continually reinvent and reinvigorate ourselves. I love working for start-ups and educating myself on each aspect of development. I've been able to complete the career level tracks in user experience and design, back- and front-end development, digital marketing, Python, analytical chemistry, and deep learning. I've reinvented myself many times as a relief physician, computer programmer, user design expert, network medical anchor, war correspondent, TV host, motor learning architect, exercise physiologist, and even sponsored professional surfer.

ONLINE PLATFORMS

You may have delayed continuing education because you thought you required one or two years of school and a new master's degree.

Online learning has turned education on its head, with extremely detailed and high-quality instruction across a huge number of subjects at extremely attractive prices. Let's look at some of the most popular learning platforms:

The Price Revolution: Daunted by the price of a $3,000 online university course or a $30,000 degree? The price revolution has made learning available to everyone worldwide, from the Upper Nile in Egypt and war-torn Syria to rural North Dakota. The price? As little as $9.99 a course. Ambitious students can become real experts and get jobs spending just a few hundred dollars. These courses often have a preview, so you can determine if the course holds interest for you or not before you invest. For many of us sitting on the sidelines, contemplating studying a new subject, these astonishing new platforms remove nearly all the barriers. Not enough background in a subject? You can go back to the very basics and work your way up .

Platform 1: Udemy, Inc.: This is the Wild West of online learning. As an example, once I took the Stanford and Coursera courses on deep learning, I was left thinking there has to be much more to this field. So many platforms have an introductory level that leaves you without enough education to make a career change or use the subject in your current career. However, www.udemy.com has hundreds of advanced deep learning courses that are just spectacular. And the number of students is just astounding. Hundreds of thousands. What I love is that so many ambitious young kids around the world who don't have the opportunity to go to a great college or get into a computer science course can complete these courses and get real jobs. The quality is variable and sometimes hard to understand, but on average they are fabulous. Just be a discerning buyer. Many courses include the actual computer code, so you can check your answers to make certain you are writing the correct computer code given in the homework assignments. Packt Publishing and udemy.com often have code to go with their courses.

Example 1: Deep learning: The most breathtaking development across most of business, academia, and science is the advent of deep learning, the heart of much artificial intelligence. I embarked on mastering this subject in order to apply it to medicine and my various projects. The artificial neural network is the heart of artificial intelligence. However, before diving into deep neural networks, it's vital to understand the mathematical background.

Matrix Algebra: Yep! Took it again. An artificial neural network forms the heart of many deep learning solutions. Deep learning, in turn, is at the core of much artificial intellegence. The form used to enter data into these networks is termed a matrix. Matrix Alegebra teaches you how to do the math required.

Differential Calculus: Defining the point at which there is the least amount of loss error (called loss) is determined by differential calculus. You don't actually have to do it yourself, unless you are programming from the ground up; however, understanding differential calculus will give you greater insights into the core of deep learning, since it is the determination of the smallest amount of error that allows the neural networks to work.

Power libraries: Writing you own neural networks from the ground up is a daunting task. However, a number of applications do some or all of the heavy lifting for you, writing huge sections of the code in specialized libraries you can call on. Great to understand the matrix algebra and differential calculus, but no need to do it yourself.

Keras: This is the most widely used library for deep learning. It allows you to construct a neural network in just a very few lines of code. When I first learned to code, it was in assembler language and Fortran. Using machine language, I might have written hundreds of lines of code. With Keras, it's less than ten lines!

Deep learning: Here are a few of the courses I took. Have a look at both the tremendous variety and at the tremendous depth of knowledge reflected in these choices. Being "bilingual" becomes a tremendous asset. That is, knowing deep learning plus your profession:

The Complete Neural Networks Bootcamp
Deep Learning A-Z
Practical Deep Learning with Keras
Practical Deep Learning with PyTorch
Building Deep Neural Networks in Keras
The Complete Python Course for Machine Learning
Scikit-Learn in Python for Machine Learning Engineers
Artificial Intelligence #5: MLP Networks
Mathematical Model for Deep Learning
Learn Java Crash Course
Complete Python Bootcamp
Deep Learning with Python and Keras
Feature Selection for Machine Learning
Build Neural Networks in Seconds
Complete Linear Algebra for Deep Learning
Hands-on Machine Learning with Python
Complete Data Visualization
Applied Machine Learning
Python for Data Science and Deep Learning
Machine Learning
Deep Learning Visual Exploration

Example 2: Write your first symphony: Sound preposterous? My whole life, I've always wanted to write a symphony but simply had no concept as to how I could write one. I began taking an online course on music composition, and learned I just needed to come up with one key musical idea, called a motif ... just a measure or two. More advanced courses teach you how to embellish that motif by extending, contracting, and moving the motif up and down. After taking two dozen courses, some of which are below, I bought a Korg Kronos workstation and mastered several of the notation software programs that allow a composer to directly input the notes into the score. I learned Sibelius, Notion, and MuseScore online. I can only imagine how many hundreds more pieces Mozart would have written with the new technology! He had dozens of scribes copying orchestral parts in his day. Bach had to write twenty-five minutes of music a week, a Herculean task when you have to transcribe all the individual instrumental parts by hand. Today, you can press a button, and the notation software prints out the entire score with each individual orchestral instrument part! I'm quickly finding out if I have the talent to compose. Since I'm interested in classical music, I play the wonderful new streaming service Idagio all day long to listen to the very best performances. This service has the highest-quality recordings of all the major conductors. The BBC also has a wonderful series of documentaries on each of the major classical composers and conductors, with tremendous insights to inspire you. Here are some music courses I took online; the fee was $9.99 for many of them:

Music

Music Composition with the Piano

Music Theory Comprehensive

Music Composition 1-14

Music Composition 2

Orchestration

Compose Orchestral Music

The Complete Piano and Music Theory Course

Platform 2: Lynda.com has a broad range of in-depth courses that are extremely clear and professionally done. The bite-sized lessons allow you to do one on the way to work and another on the way home. I click on a Lynda lesson instead of surfing on my iPhone. You'll find great satisfaction in completing a few chapters every day. They are as short as two minutes and as long as nine minutes. If you have curiosity about an area, just watch the introductory video on a subject. The fee is $19.99 monthly for a year. Below are some of the 322 courses I've taken:

Music

Music: Sibelius 8 Essential Training
Music Theory for Songwriters
Introduction to Songwriting
Pro Tools 11 Essential Training
Learning Songwriting

Artificial Intelligence

Explainable Artificial Intelligence
Python: Programming Efficiently
Learning Java
Building and Deploying Deep Learning Applications with TensorFlow
Building Deep Learning Applications with Keras 2.0
Designing for Neural Networks and AI Interfaces
Designing an Onboarding Experience with InVision and Sketch
Learning Python with PyCharm
MATLAB 2018 Essential Training
Artificial Intelligence Foundations: Neural Networks
Data Science Foundations
Neural Networks and Convolutional Networks Essential Training
Learning Python
Machine Learning and AI Foundations: Classification Modeling
Data Science and Analytics Career Paths
Data Science Foundations: Python Scientific Stack
Machine Learning and AI Foundations: Predictive Modeling Strategy
    at Scale
Python Statistics Essential Training
Accelerating TensorFlow with Google Machine Learning
Machine Learning and AI Foundations: Clustering
Machine Learning and AI Foundations: Linear Regression
Data Science Foundations: Data Mining
Drawing Vector Graphics
Sketch for UX Design

User design sits at the interface between the user and the technical code under the hood of every major platform, from Uber to Airbnb. The quality of the user experience determines how easy the platform is to use—and the likability! Here are some of the courses I took to understand the process and to be part of the discussion in various tech start-ups where I'm invited to help.

Sketch: This program allows you to quickly design a screen that can then be ported from desktop to iPad to iPhone to Android with ease.

InVision Essential Training: This genius program allows designers to link user screens to create a working user experience for testing. InVision Studio First Look pulls design and screen linkage into one platform.

Platform 3: Packt:[76] This platform is great for deep learning. What I like about it is that you have actual books to read, lessons you can watch, and code you can download. Here's what I've done recently:

Deep Learning
Music Composition
User Design and Experience

Example 3: Learn a new language: Prologue: "Islis ijlis, kateer jiddan!" "Sit down, it's dangerous!" I yelled in Arabic, crouching in a long ditch with a 14-year-old girl clutching her baby while we tracked an overhead fusillade of mortar and gunfire between the US Marines and the fedayeen outside of Al-Kūt during the invasion of Iraq.

Soon the gunfire let up and, as we saw in the previous chapter, the Marine colonel shouted at me: "Bob, do you want to bring our guests in for lunch?"

I scrambled through the Marine lines carrying the baby, then sat with her. "Tureedeen an taakalee—lahm dijaj au lahm bakar?" "Which do you prefer to eat, chicken or fish?" I asked.

"Chicken," she said.

---

76 www.packtpub.com

Then the fedayeen started firing at us. To recount the story, two Bell AH-1 Cobra helicopters spun up and started firing TOW missiles at their positions. The girl, baby, and I ran up to the top of an incline, where three M1A1 tanks had just arrived. Providing cover, we stood behind the tanks. I took the microphone over to the Marine Colonel.

"Colonel, you have heavy incoming machine gun fire, your Humvee was almost hit, an RPG landed just yards away. What do you have to say?"

He stood ramrod straight, looked into the camera, and said, "It's a great day to be a US Marine!"

What a great moment! Would never have been there without learning Arabic!!!

As a lifelong humanitarian, I find no greater satisfaction than being able to assist the most desperate while communicating with them in their own language. I've always loved languages; I have mastered some and picked up bits and pieces of others. I'm not a natural linguist and have to learn them by brute force. I began with German, spending a year at the University of Innsbruck, and I continued with French during a semester at the University of Fribourg in Switzerland. I began learning Arabic at the Sana'a Institute for the Arabic Language in Yemen and Swahili at the Institute of Kiswahili and Foreign Languages in Zanzibar. The others I picked up from books and practice during reporting, competition, or humanitarian trips in Kosovo, Japan, Zimbabwe, Botswana, and Norway.

Languages and aging: Psycholinguist Mark Antoniou of Western Sydney University in Australia suggested "... that multiple-language use on a regular basis may help delay the onset of Alzheimer's disease."

Here are the key reasons language helps, according to Mark:

1. It improves executive function. "[It] allows you to control, direct, and manage your attention, as well as your ability to plan. It also helps you ignore irrelevant information and focus on what's important."[77]

---

77 https://www.knowablemagazine.org/article/mind/2018/how-second-language-can-boost-brain

2. It improves brain structure, creating denser gray matter and more high-functioning white matter with better, more highly functioning connections.

It's great to start as a child, but newer research shows you can learn languages as an adult and benefit. Let's look at how:

HOW TO LEARN A NEW LANGUAGE

Grammar: Sure, we hated grammar as kids, but it really is the secret behind learning language, because grammar gives you a game plan. Once you know some grammar, you can use a limited vocabulary in a robust number of ways. As an example, you could learn one verb, then deploy it in first, second, or third person, past, present, or future. This makes you sound quite educated and inflates one word into a dozen or more uses!

Strategy

Get a clear answer: Employ an offensive strategy as you start speaking, since you may put together some pretty nice sentences but have no idea what the respondent may say as they rattle off at high speed in a dialect that's really foreign to you. So, make a statement, then ask a question that warrants yes or no!

Ask for help correcting errors. Studies show that you often learn best through error corrections. Many of us are reluctant to speak a foreign language because we'll look stupid or embarrass ourselves. Not at all! Throw it all out there. Just ask for help. When others correct your error, you'll create the strongest memory link. Years later, I can recall where I properly learned how to use a verb. In Khartoum in the Nineties, during one of the many wars and crises there, I asked my driver not to hit the truck bearing down on us. He corrected my use of the verb yatasaddam which is "to collide." I remember to this day the emphasis and doubling the Ds in the middle!

How I learn

The basics: First I buy a good grammar book, then I memorize 100 verbs and 1,000 nouns. Then I start to inflict myself on anyone who will listen, ask for corrections, and try to absorb the corrections.

Fluency: As we begin learning languages, brain scans show us using huge parts of our brain. But as language becomes more automatic, we use smaller and smaller parts, until we're fully fluent. What a wonderful feeling this accomplishment is! As you read in the motor learning chapter, this process is remarkably similar to learning a new sport.

Platforms

Rosetta Stone: This is a great way to start hearing and pronouncing the language. Academics fault Rosetta Stone for not having grammar, which is quite hard to deduce. However, the program will develop your ear and pronunciation by helping to correct your accent. The examples are not always practical, and you won't learn basic survival communications in the first lessons.

Rocket Languages: This is a more stripped-down platform but still decent for picking up vocabulary.

Google Translate: Fabulous tool! Think of what you want to say, and Google translates to over 100 languages. I'll respond to Instagram posts in dozens of languages I don't know a word of! Fun! Just hope it's accurate so that it doesn't start a small conflict in some remote corner of the planet! I also love the pronunciation the platform does for you!

Live tutors: I've had huge successes getting tutored. Now there are wonderful services that allow you to hire a tutor by the hour and take the lessons via Skype!

Varsity Tutors: "Bob! Jim here. Do you think you could record a commercial in French? Quebecois French?" Varsity Tutors was incredibly professional, calling me immediately and lining up a tutor for the following day. They sell reasonable packages of fifteen lessons.

I had a language emergency and pressed the ASAP function on their site. I had a live tutor ten minutes later who was incredibly helpful, skilled, and intelligent. For the final preparation I used a dialect expert who coached me in the finer points of Quebecois, the French spoken in Quebec.

Wyzant: This online service has 8,000 tutors, many available on short notice. Try to find a tutor who works well for you. I find there are certain styles that work best for me. I prefer to have predetermined vocabularies, so the tutor is using words I know and I'm not trying to guess meanings of new words. Tutors are also so valuable for pronouncing difficult words.

Joy Jukes: Joy is a fabulous dialect coach when you need to perfect your accent for the movies!

Books: Teach Yourself series: I always loved this series, which has a simple format with great examples. Teach Yourself usually has separate grammar and vocabulary books for major languages like French. I underline these books and keep them on a shelf. I might not speak a language for years, but when I need to, I spend a few days reviewing my underlining, and I'm ready to go. For instance, I have an upcoming trip to Eastern Congo. I've dusted off my Teach Yourself Swahili book and am rememorizing all the vocabulary I've underlined.

Language philosophy

Decide on the usefulness of particular language before embarking on learning it. For instance, I love Norwegian and have studied it in Beitostølen during the Masters World Cup cross-country skiing championships, but there is no Norwegian that doesn't speak flawless English, and so it has no practical use outside of Norway (with crossover in Sweden, where you could make yourself understood.) However, you can deploy Spanish through the Western Hemisphere and Europe.

My other philosophy in learning multiple languages is to pick very different languages from different geographical areas. The benefit to this concept is that the languages will be different enough that you won't confuse them—Italian, French, and Spanish have a lot of crossover, but Arabic and German don't!

Here's what I've studied:

Africa: Swahili, Shona
Europe: German, French
Asia: Japanese, Mandarin
Middle East: Arabic

MILLENNIAL LEARNING

My millennial son's friends often ask me about career direction. I'll send them a note with suggested courses they can preview to determine if it's an interest. Should they like the preview, I encourage them to take a few courses on Udemy to see if they are interested. When they find courses of interest they excel in, then they can dig in, learning enough for a career switch.

MID-CAREER LEARNING

I work with a code academy in Vermont. Their market is mid-career, looking at people who want to shift to a new career. In as little as twelve weeks they have a completely new skill in coding, with a 93 percent employment rate and an average starting salary of $73,000! Never think it's too late to embrace a new career. I had a producer at CBS News, Lisa Sanders, who decided at age 39 she wanted to pursue medicine. She completed two years of pre-med at Columbia, then enrolled at Yale to study medicine.

RETIREMENT LEARNING

I see many retirees taking broad general interest courses. I don't believe in that. If you're 65, you have at least ten years of life expectancy, perhaps twenty. Use the time to get really good at one or two subjects. Work hard and you are a world-class expert by 75. Sure, take general courses to see if you have an interest or could develop one, but then advance in that area as far as you can. You'll be so much more energized and inspirational when you talk with others. Being up to speed on the newest technologies like machine learning also helps erase the age gap, so you can have dynamic, fun conversations with millennials and centennials! I love meeting my college-aged son's friends and chatting about Python or constructing deep learning networks.

PART V:

BATTLE

"Aging is not for the faint of heart," said actor George Clooney, referring to his life on screen.

Fighting the aging process is an epic, life-or-death battle. I don't want to mislead you into believing that if you stay fit and eat a great diet, you'll avoid all of life's maladies. Chances are you won't. That's why you should place the epic battle against chronic illness at the forefront of staying young. How aggressively you react to risk and illness determines how you age and how long you live. The biggest villain is now called polymorbidity—not just one but several chronic conditions on the attack. You have to fight illness with dogged persistence. In modern medicine there is little to no follow-up after medical visits. You're therefore left to wallow on your own, so you'll have to aggressively chart your own course, assessing all of your risk factors and attacking them one by one. Beginning in your twenties, you'll want to mount an aggressive attack on key risk factors, ranging from binge drinking and obesity to the increasing risks of heart disease, anxiety, and depression. By your forties, the first signs of real disease begin. In your fifties, the battle begins. In your sixties and seventies, the battle rages, and you are in a fight for your life.

I counsel many patients about battle and push them hard to fight each battle when it's a small brush fire and not a raging inferno. Senior Dartmouth-Hitchcock cardiologist Jon Wahrenberger counseled me that so many chronic illnesses, manageable on their own, coalesce to simply overwhelm the patient. The patient simply gives up, grows old, and dies. Be forewarned! Don't let this happen to you. We in the media have made preventive health care seem easy. It's not. Disease is complex, and you will want a first-rate team to mount an assault on each and every malady at the onset.

What will your future be? Remember watching the movie A Christmas Carol as a kid? Wasn't the scene terrifying when Scrooge's partner, Joseph Marley, reappears from the dead as the Ghost of Christmas Past? Entrapped by chains and enveloped by gloom, Joseph warns Scrooge about a Christmas yet to come. Well, there are two visions of yourself in the years yet to come:

Vision 1: Defeated and humbled by decades of abuse, disuse, and illness, surrendering to middle and old age as you become a burden to others.

Vision 2: Life as a youthful 25-year-old for decades beyond your most optimistic expectations and serving as an inspiration to all.

Since a huge and under-recognized piece of beating the aging process is how you battle the onslaught of chronic illnesses that befall all of us, I tried to imagine what life would have been like without taking full advantage of all modern medicine. Here's what Dr. Bob would look like without aggressively battling chronic illness and just letting warnings, prominent risk factors, and symptoms slide. To make the contrast starker, I've set the comparison between 1920 and the present. Even today, the vast majority of Americans live as they did a century ago, allowing many of these afflictions to overwhelm and doom them. As you'll observe, modern medicine has become the greatest miracle of our time, helping us overcome hundreds of illnesses and conditions that would have killed or crippled us in the past.

Arthritis 1920: I'd have been confined to a wheelchair, at best taking a few steps with a walker, in tremendous pain and growing fat from inactivity.
   Cause: Severe "bone on bone" arthritis of the hips, untreatable in 1920.

Arthritis 2020: A genius hip-resurfacing operation allows me to compete in the 32-mile world championship between two islands in

Hawaii on a narrow paddleboard in giant oceans. Instead of hobbling on a walker, I compete in 50-kilometer cross-country ski marathons during the winter and race giant slalom. Many Americans today delay for years the joint replacement surgery that could restore their mobility. I couldn't walk two blocks before this operation. I'll take you through the steps of deciding when to consider joint replacement.

Lung disease 1920: I'd be coughing up mounds of dark green and yellow sputum while wheezing into a primitive home oxygen system throughout the day and night. My nights would be spent waking every hour to fits of coughing up mounds of sputum out of my lungs and into a bucket. Super-tight airways and increasingly severe asthma would make life terrifying, with an ever-increasing sense of doom.

    Cause: Asthma and bronchiectasis

Lung disease 2020: Inhaled steroids, antibiotics, lung physical therapy, sinus surgery, esophageal surgery, and bronchodilators give me a symptom-free life with an occasional cough and modest symptoms of asthma.

Gastroesophageal reflux (heartburn) 1920: Severe heartburn would have made every hour wretched, pouring acid and pepsin into my lungs and sinuses and onto my vocal cords. I'd never enjoy a meal and would be too hoarse to speak in more than a whisper. I'd have a nearly constant searing feel of acid snaking up my esophagus.

    Cause: Gastroesophageal reflux, where acid from the stomach surges back into your esophagus and up into your lungs and sinuses.

Gastroesophageal reflux 2020: During 2017, I lay awake every night, coughing and hacking on a veterinary dose of antibiotics, steroids, and inhalers without enough. A once draconian procedure called a Nissen fundoplication corrects the defect that causes reflux. The Lap Nissen is now a minimally invasive technique taking four and a half hours under general anesthesia. Genius surgeon Ted Trus,

MD, performed this surgery on me at Dartmouth-Hitchcock Medical Center. I woke up in recovery with only a minimal residual cough. After a night in the hospital, I was back in the gym the next day. Six months later, my symptoms have vanished. I had considered a top Harvard hospital, but Dartmouth's chair of medicine, Rich Rothstein, MD, took me aside and said, "Ted is just as good a surgeon, and you will have a much better experience!" Boy, did I!!! Fantastic personnel made the hospital stay a joy.

Sinusitis 1920: Chronically infected sinuses trigger worsened lung disease and lead to constant headaches and a complete loss of smell. If the ability to do a CT scan existed back then, my lungs would have looked like a fine Swiss cheese, with acid eating away at the small airways.

    Cause: Reflux from the stomach, up the esophagus, and into the sinuses caused raging sinus inflammation and infection.

Sinusitis today: In 2018, minimally invasive surgery cleared out the blockages in the sinuses and cleaned out the infection. I awoke from this two-hour procedure with my cough gone! (With the return of symptoms in 2019, brilliant ENT surgeon Sarah Seo operated on my ethmoidal and sphenoidal sinuses; 90 percent of my cough was gone within a week.)

Heart 1920: My coronary arteries would have filled with sludge. I'd have suffered multiple heart attacks, and I would have had very little function left.

    Cause: Extremely high-fat diets were the rule and accelerated coronary artery disease. No doctor had even dreamed of a medication. Even in the Fifties, heart attacks were treated with oxygen and bed rest.

Heart 2020: A calcium test showed extensive calcium in my coronary arteries. Blood tests showed high inflammation and high bad cholesterol. A terrific high polyphenol diet and cholesterol-lowering drugs left me completely free of any symptoms of heart disease. Yet today, a terrible diet and toxic lifestyles are the leading cause of the heart, diabetes, and obesity epidemics.

Cataracts 1920: I would have been unable to read, work jigsaw puzzles, collect stamps, button my shirt, or find my zipper.
Cause: Nearly completely opacified cataracts prevented reading any detail.

Cataracts 2020: Cataract surgery, which seems so mundane today, has restored me to better than perfect vision, 20/15 in each eye. I have better vision than a teenager!

"Geez," you might say. "Dr. Bob, you're a mess! So many illnesses." Well, I should be a mess, but I'm not. I live nearly symptom free from a host of chronic illnesses by aggressively pursuing the best medical care from a range of specialists. Honestly, though, I had no idea it would be so challenging and cause so much pain! I thought I'd sail through my 70s, instead I've threaded through some very rocky shoals in a full gale! Be tough. Track down each sign and symptom. Get solid diagnoses and pursue each illness relentlessly. For instance, many patients would be satisfied with a diagnosis of chronic obstructive disease. A more through probing might have found, as in my case, that 90 percent of the illness came from infected sinuses and esophageal reflux. With removal of the esophagus and sinuses, my lung disease began to vanish, as revealed on a CT scan.

Modern medicine is an astonishing miracle for those who take great care of themselves and take it to its maximum benefit. Chronic illness will take its toll if treated casually. Tragically, too many of us live as we might have in 1918, passively allowing a range of maladies to overwhelm us.

Like an old car falling apart, there's not just one fault as we age. Wear and tear on the engine, shocks, tires, transmission, bumpers, and body cause a car to age, but restore each element, and it runs like new. Aggressively pursuing each part of your health is a huge piece of turning back the clock and grasping youth from the bony hands of the grim reaper!

I've been blessed with fantastic medical providers at Dartmouth-Hitchcock Medical Center (DHMC), the Hospital for Special Surgery (HSS), and Stowe Family Practice. Dartmouth's Rick Enelow, MD, has proven a fantastic strategist, finding each of these nuanced conditions and linking me with the right tests, procedures, and surgeries. Dartmouth's chair of medicine, Rich Rothstein, MD, has proven to be a medical mastermind in his fantastic overview of my illnesses and in pointing me toward major surgery as a final fix for my worst nightmare. As the slogan goes, don't look where doctors refer patients, look where they get their own care. I love the care I get at Dartmouth. As Rich told me: "Bob, we are just as good as the care you will receive at Harvard, you'll just have a much better experience." I certainly have. DHMC feels like family. The whole staff makes me feel incredibly welcome and like they really care for me. HSS, as we'll see, gets the best results in the world for orthopedic diseases, and it's where I go and where I refer orthopedic cases, especially joint replacement. Our local Stowe Family Practice has been fantastic at determining the basic risks and vaccine strategies. Very thankful to Clea James, MD, and her whole team!

Complexity

I'm overawed still by how complex medicine is, and how incredibly difficult it is to get the right diagnosis and treatment. Many of us suffer and age far more quickly with the burden of chronic illness. This can be easy to manage in your twenties and thirties but may appear nearly impossible to address with advancing age. The media can portray medicine as an easy plug-and-play:

High cholesterol? Take a statin!
High cholesterol? Take a water pill (diuretic)!!
Acid Reflux? Take a Zantac!!!

Risk assessment

An individual assessment of your actual risks is vital to determining an overarching strategy. I have a patient who was overweight. Her friends played medical experts and counseled her regularly to lose weight and improve her diet. In the end, that routine advice was just plain wrong. Her key risk was smoking, which outweighed all others. This put her at risk of a brain aneurysm, which she did suffer. A smoking cessation program and blood pressure monitoring would have been a far more effective strategy.

I had another patient who was lean and athletic, and who carefully watched his diet. He suffered heartburn for years and treated it with Tums and over-the-counter remedies. He developed early esophageal cancer. More careful tracking of this esophageal cancer risk and definitive treatment with prescription medications and regular endoscopy would have uncovered this condition when it was pre-cancerous. So, look hard at your own individual risks and not at what pop culture sends your way!

Heart disease remains the number-one risk over time. While you may be fine at 50 or 60, you may die of heart disease at 85, since it remains a progressive disease. One of the worst unforced errors is believing that being in top cardiovascular shape, even as a competitive athlete, somehow makes you immune to heart disease. It doesn't, researchers at the University of British Columbia report. They determined that even the fittest Master athletes are not immune to cardiovascular disease. Worse still, they often don't have any symptoms. I know! I achieved the highest level in a stress test, better than 99.99 percent of men in my age group, yet a coronary CT showed severe disease. This got my attention, and I embarked upon a very aggressive preventive program, including statins and baby aspirin. The study followed 798 "Master athletes"—adults aged 35 and older who engaged in moderate-to-vigorous physical activity at least three days a week. The participants included a range of athletes—runners, cyclists, triathletes, rowers, and hockey players.

Those with risk factors took a stress test, and then those with evidence of disease went on to a CT coronary angiogram to determine if they had cardiovascular disease.

Of the 798 athletes, ninety-four (11 percent) were found to have significant cardiovascular disease. Ten participants were found to have severe coronary artery disease (a blockage in their artery of 70 percent or greater), despite not having any symptoms.

See a cardiologist for a full evaluation. Get checked for high blood pressure, high cholesterol, inflammation, and a family history of cardiovascular disease.

Although the noninvasive CT stress test remains somewhat controversial, I'm a huge fan for one reason. If you have no calcium, there's likely no reason to undergo cholesterol-lowering therapy. However, a high calcium score suggests that statin therapy may be a good option.

Stress test with echocardiogram

A well-performed stress test with an echocardiogram is just a terrific way to be sure you can go to your highest heart rate without chest pain, problems with the beating wall of your heart, or exercise-provoked irregular heartbeats. I had one performed recently at Dartmouth-Hitchcock Medical Center. I asked how many of their clients ended up going to ICU. They said around 20 percent. So, for these patients, the stress test made a ton of sense. Even though I was in great shape, it just made sense to be sure I was really safe. And I was! A well-performed stress test looks at each of your heart valves, the wall motion of your heart, how much blood is being pumped out, and how much of your maximum predicted heart rate you can reach before exhaustion sets in. It's a great, safe test. The key is to be very aggressive about lowering your cholesterol and inflammation levels. If you're going to live into your mid-eighties, coronary artery disease is going to slowly creep up on you, so you'll want to be extremely aggressive about achieving low levels of LDL—well below 100—and low levels of inflammation.

Calculating Global CHD Risk in Men

Step 1: Age

Years	Points	Years	Points
30 to 34	-1	55 to 59	4
35 to 39	0	60 to 64	5
40 to 44	1	65 to 69	6
45 to 49	2	70 to 74	7
50 to 54	3		

Step 2: LDL or TC Level

LDL		
mg per dL	mmol per L	Points
< 100	< 2.59	-3
100 to 129	2.59 to 3.35	0
130 to 159	3.36 to 4.13	0
160 to 190	4.14 to 4.92	1
> 190	> 4.92	2

TC		
mg per dL	mmol per L	Points
< 160	< 4.14	-3
160 to 199	4.14 to 5.16	0
200 to 239	5.17 to 6.20	1
240 to 279	6.21 to 7.23	2
≥ 280	≥ 7.24	3

Step 3: HDL Level

mg per dL	mmol per L	Points (if LDL used in step 2)	Points (if TC used in step 2)
< 35	< 0.91	2	2
35 to 44	0.91 to 1.15	1	1
45 to 49	1.16 to 1.28	0	0
50 to 59	1.29 to 1.54	0	0
≥ 60	≥ 1.55	-1	-2

Step 4: Blood Pressure

Systolic (mm Hg)	Diastolic (mm Hg)				
	< 80	80 to 84	85 to 89	90 to 99	≥ 100
< 120	0 points				
120 to 129		0 points			
130 to 139			1 point		
140 to 159				2 points	
≥ 160					3 points

NOTE: When systolic and diastolic pressures provide different point scores, use the higher score.

Step 5: Diabetes Mellitus

Present?	Points
No	0
Yes	2

Step 6: Smoking

Smoker?	Points
No	0
Yes	2

Step 7: Total Points

Step 1: Age	___
Step 2: LDL or TC level	___
Step 3: HDL level	___
Step 4: Blood pressure	___
Step 5: Diabetes mellitus	___
Step 6: Smoking	___
Total points	___

Step 8: CHD Risk

Total points	10-year risk if LDL used in step 2 (%)	10-year risk if TC used in step 2 (%)
≤ -3	1	—
-2	2	—
-1	2	2
0	3	3
1	4	3
2	4	4
3	6	5
4	7	7
5	9	8
6	11	10
7	14	13
8	18	16
9	22	20
10	27	25
11	33	31
12	40	37
13	47	45
≥ 14	≥ 56	≥ 53

Step 9: Comparative Risk

Age (years)	Average 10-year CHD risk (%)	Average 10-year risk of hard event* (%)	Low 10-year CHD risk† (%)
30 to 34	3	1	2
35 to 39	5	4	3
40 to 44	7	4	4
45 to 49	11	8	4
50 to 54	14	10	6
55 to 59	16	13	7
60 to 64	21	20	9
65 to 69	25	22	11
70 to 74	30	25	14

*—Hard events exclude angina pectoris.
†—Low risk as calculated for a man of the same age who does not smoke or have diabetes, and has optimal blood pressure, an LDL level of 100 to 129 mg per dL or TC level of 160 to 199 mg per dL, and an HDL level of 45 mg per dL.

Key

Color	Relative risk	Color	Relative risk
Green	Very low	Orange	High
White	Low	Red	Very high
Yellow	Moderate		

Calculating Global CHD Risk in Women

Step 1: Age

Years	Points	Years	Points
30 to 34	-9	55 to 59	7
35 to 39	-4	60 to 64	8
40 to 44	0	65 to 69	8
45 to 49	3	70 to 74	8
50 to 54	6		

Step 2: LDL or TC Level

LDL

mg per dL	mmol per L	Points
< 100	< 2.59	-2
100 to 129	2.59 to 3.35	0
130 to 159	3.36 to 4.13	0
160 to 190	4.14 to 4.92	2
> 190	> 4.92	2

TC

mg per dL	mmol per L	Points
< 160	< 4.14	-2
160 to 199	4.14 to 5.16	0
200 to 239	5.17 to 6.20	1
240 to 279	6.21 to 7.23	1
≥ 280	≥ 7.24	3

Step 3: HDL Level

mg per dL	mmol per L	Points (if LDL used in step 2)	Points (if TC used in step 2)
< 35	< 0.91	5	5
35 to 44	0.91 to 1.15	2	2
45 to 49	1.16 to 1.28	1	1
50 to 59	1.29 to 1.54	0	0
≥ 60	≥ 1.55	-2	-3

Step 4: Blood Pressure

Systolic (mm Hg)	Diastolic (mm Hg)				
	< 80	80 to 84	85 to 89	90 to 99	≥ 100
< 120	-3 points				
120 to 129		0 points			
130 to 139			0 points		
140 to 159				2 points	
≥ 160					3 points

NOTE: When systolic and diastolic pressures provide different point scores, use the higher score.

Step 5: Diabetes Mellitus

Present?	Points
No	0
Yes	4

Step 6: Smoking

Smoker?	Points
No	0
Yes	2

Step 7: Total Points

Step 1: Age	___
Step 2: LDL or TC level	___
Step 3: HDL level	___
Step 4: Blood pressure	___
Step 5: Diabetes mellitus	___
Step 6: Smoking	___
Total points	___

Step 8: CHD Risk

Total points	10-year risk if LDL used in step 2 (%)	10-year risk if TC used in step 2 (%)
≤ -2	1	1
-1	2	2
0	2	2
1	2	2
2	3	3
3	3	3
4	4	4
5	5	4
6	6	5
7	7	6
8	8	7
9	9	8
10	11	10
11	13	11
12	15	13
13	17	15
14	20	18
15	24	20
16	27	24
≥ 17	≥ 32	≥ 27

Step 9: Comparative Risk

Age (years)	Average 10-year CHD risk (%)	Average 10-year risk of hard event* (%)	Low 10-year CHD risk† (%)
30 to 34	< 1	< 1	< 1
35 to 39	< 1	< 1	1
40 to 44	2	1	2
45 to 49	5	2	3
50 to 54	8	3	5
55 to 59	12	7	7
60 to 64	12	8	8
65 to 69	13	8	8
70 to 74	14	11	8

*—Hard events exclude angina pectoris.
†—Low risk as calculated for a woman of the same age who does not smoke or have diabetes, and has optimal blood pressure; an LDL level of 100 to 129 mg per dL or TC level of 160 to 199 mg per dL, and an HDL level of 55 mg per dL (1.42 mmol per L).

Key

Color	Relative risk	Color	Relative risk
Green	Very low	Orange	High
White	Low	Red	Very high
Yellow	Moderate		

Get world-class care

In reality, medicine is incredibly complex, as we have just seen. Here's what I recommend.

1. Find a world-class medical center close to you. Here are my choices:

    Massachusetts General Hospital: simply the finest hospital in the world with sub-sub specialists for every imaginable condition. Physicians and surgeons have an insatiable curiosity about illness. As MGH President Peter Slavin says, "Illness is the enemy!"

    New York Presbyterian: I have referred hundreds of the most complex cardiac surgeries to Wayne Isom and his colleagues and have always been astounded by the spectacular results.

    The Hospital for Special Surgery: This is where I refer nearly all my joint-replacement and orthopedic patients. I've had my own hips resurfaced there.

    UCLA: Fantastic referrals to a wide range of expert sub-sub specialists

    Dartmouth-Hitchcock Medical Center: The greatest jewel found in a small and easily accessible medical center.

    US News & World Report rates medical centers nationwide and is a decent place to start.

2. Find a strategist at one of these hospitals and stick with him or her. Assess all your risks and symptoms. Track them down relentlessly. In modern medicine, specialists have a single-minded focus and will be fantastic at solving highly specific problems. However, a strategist will have an overview that will see, as an example, that asthma, reflux disease, sinusitis, and inflammation leading to heart disease are part of one big puzzle that needs to be solved.

3. Seek early definitive care. For instance, with atrial fibrillation,

look at ablative treatment as soon as you are eligible. This erases the underling aberrant electrical pathways that cause AF. Modern surgery is so low risk that I'm a huge fan of tackling problems early and aggressively. I've had these surgeries, each of which has made an immeasurable improvement in my life:

Cataract removal and new lens insertion
Hernia repair
Esophageal repair (Nissen)
Hip resurfacing
Sinus surgery

Humans naturally procrastinate in undertaking diagnostic tests and medical procedures. Modern teams and anesthetics make surgery a very pleasant experience, as does pain management. Charge headlong at whatever maladies you suffer for an early and successful outcome.

4. Look for great outcomes. You can further hone your search by looking for the outcomes of individual practitioners. For instance, for bypass surgery, you'll want a death rate even for a complicated case at 1 percent or less.

Follow these steps and you'll shortcut an accelerating aging process and vastly improve your quality of life.

Managing pain

Several years ago, I approached the M2O world championship with a great deal of trepidation and pain. This grueling stand-up paddling race covers thirty-two miles of the most dangerous ocean on earth. In desperation, I took five ibuprofen tablets before the start. Soon my stomach started to hurt, then it really hurt. I started to retch. Doubled over in pain, I lay down on the board, hoping the pain would go away. Like many older athletes who have some medical ailments and are taking a variety of medications, adding oral pain therapy can be a disaster. We may take them like candy, but these have serious short- and long-term consequences. Let's look at them by the numbers.

Ibuprofen: There are 16,500 deaths from ibuprofen usage each year. The FDA has warned that there is a 10-50 percent increase in the risk of heart attack and stroke, depending on the doses and length of time these are ingested. Take ibuprofen only for limited periods of time. If you are constantly sore and taking ibuprofen every day, you're over-trained and need to back off. If you have joint pain after exercise, you risk damaging the joints by continuing to pound on them with the aid of pain relievers rather than letting them recover. I take a Zantac with ibuprofen to decrease the risk of stomach bleeding, should taking it be a necessity.

Acetaminophen: There are 450 deaths annually. Though thought of as the safe alternative, an overdose is the leading cause of liver failure in the US, leading to the need for a liver transplant. There are 50,000 ER visits and 25,000 hospitalizations. Be sure to limit yourself to less than 4 grams a day from all sources. Many combination medications contain acetaminophen, so that you may unintentionally exceed this limit. Multiple high doses are even more dangerous for heavy drinkers.

Opioids: Over 17,000 Americans die annually from overdosing on prescribed opioids. All opioids combined total 47,000 deaths. The head of the US Armed Forces Medical Service told me that soldiers with simple quad-sparing knee surgery or contusions may have been given opioids when weaker, much less addictive pain relievers might work. Also, for long-term pain, opioids are no more effective than traditional pain relievers. I had sinus surgery recently and was offered only acetaminophen. Carefully taken, I was surprised by how well they worked.

Topical pain therapy: There are zero deaths from topical pain relievers. Widely used in Germany, Singapore, and other countries, only 12.5 percent of Americans treat their pain with topical pain relievers. Yet these are the safest first choice for any pain you can touch. In medicine we say first do no harm. If you choose a topical agent first, you may start to kill chronic pain before it gets a foothold. The only significant risk is a potential skin irritation. Topical therapy is unquestionably the best therapy there is in terms of the ratio of effectiveness to danger. Topical therapy is available over the counter for about $12.95.

Compounded: These formulations hit all the key targets and can be individualized for you and the kind of pain you suffer.
Why do topicals work so well? There is a pain receptor right under your skin termed the nociceptor. This is like a switchboard for pain, with a variety of on and off switches on it. In medicine we call them receptors. Think lock and key: when the key is inserted, the pain signal is processed and sent to the brain. Most modern medications are receptor-based, blocking or activating receptors. Topical pain medications block these receptors on this pain switchboard, the nociceptor, to block pain. A famous book, Peripheral Receptor Targets for Analgesia: Novel Approaches to Pain Management by Brian E. Cairns, lays out the hundreds of different kinds of receptors, many of them potential targets for therapy. These receptors have names like mu opioid, cannabinoid, calcium-sensing, sodium, NMDA, etc. (Yes, there are real receptors that respond to cannabinoid elements.) So topical treatment works because there is great science behind it. Better still, as little as 2–15 percent of the amount you put on your skin actually gets into your bloodstream, while 24–50 times more gets to the site of the pain than when you take the same medication orally.

Prescription topicals: Many pain medications are incredibly potent but with equally powerful side effects when administered orally, by injection, or infusion. Yet these same powerful medications, like gabapentin or ketamine, given topically, go directly to the pain receptor at doses many times higher and with far fewer of the side effects. Your doctor can order a compounded pain formulation that contains several of these. The most useful ingredients include:

Ketamine
Gabapentin
Amitriptyline
Bupivacaine

OTC: Single-ingredient preparations may be bought at your local pharmacy. They have two important ingredients: an NSAID (nonsteroidal anti-inflammatory drug) and lidocaine. Salonpas has two excellent products that I use:

Salonpas Pain Relief Patch, Large: This has methyl salicylate, a key NSAID, and menthol.
Salonpas Lidocaine Plus (in cream or liquid): This has 4 percent lidocaine, the maximum amount allowed without a prescription.

I used these for the M2O race with great success.

Advice 1: Use topical pain treatment as first-line therapy. If you have more musculoskeletal pain from working out, you're better off backing off and recovering than pushing through pain with oral pain meds, since you may do real permanent harm to your joints. Consider oral meds only if topicals fail to work. Remember that simple ibuprofen can work as well as an opioid. For chronic pain, opioids prove no better than ibuprofen.

Advice 2: Keep some OTC pain products in your medicine cabinet and a fresh prescription of compounded pain formulation if you have arthritis, neuropathy, or more severe conditions, or you get regular joint or muscle pain from working out.

When to replace joints

My philosophy in my twenties was to tear through your original body parts, enjoy life to its fullest, then replace them! Of course, tempered by what I've experienced, I would employ the wisdom in the first part of this book to undertake activities with less stress on the joints! Still, the toughest decision is when to replace joints, carefully weighing the risk and benefits.

Hip: I lost all of my fifties to terrible osteoarthritis of both hips. I couldn't run or hike. By the end, I couldn't walk two city blocks. I waited far too long. Why? Sure, I worried about complications. I also knew that the later you had your hips replaced, the better chance that you'd have of avoiding a second operation, often termed a "re-do," when the original replacements fail. Total hip replacements (THR) do eventually go bad. This used to be in as little as ten to fifteen years but is now much longer. The idea was if you replace it at 65, it would last at least until you were 80. The trouble is that you would sacrifice those years while you waited.

Birmingham Hip Resurfacing (BHR): My story: Concerned about a re-do but suffering with pain all night and a major lack of mobility, I decided the time had come. My concern about the total hip replacement was that the new hips would go bad quickly due to my active lifestyle, so I was stuck deciding between a total hip replacement and BHR. I want to recall my story in detail for you in order to introduce the complex and detailed thought processes that come with making your decision.

As a television medical correspondent for decades on shows like Today, Dateline, and the CBS Evening News, and author of fourteen books on consumer medicine, I had to admit it. I never faced a more vexing decision than deciding to finally undergo a hip replacement. Even more difficult was deciding which one: a total hip replacement or a new technique called hip resurfacing, where the body's hip is left in place, but the cartilage in the socket and on all of the joint surfaces was replaced. The claims and data appeared wildly contradictory, and each surgeon's opinion was miles apart from another's. I called great friends in orthopedics at the leading Harvard hospitals and in New York, Baltimore, and Los Angeles. The word I got was emphatic:

"Don't do the hip resurfacing, it's a failed concept. It failed in the Seventies and it's doomed to fail again."

Surgeons cited a high rate of femoral fracture after the operation. They also said I could get the same advantages out of the new total hips as resurfacing—low dislocation, high activity levels, and the addition of much longer implant life than hip resurfacing. A new study from the American Academy of Orthopaedic Surgeons even showed that some of the apparent advantages of BHR were due to self-selection. Simply put, younger patients chose resurfacing, so it became a self-fulfilling prophesy: Younger patients had BHR, worked harder afterward, and did better. In other words, it wasn't the BHR, it was the self-selection.

After years of marathons, bike races, ski competitions, marathon cross-country ski races, big wall ice climbing, big wave surfing, and even accumulating a little shrapnel in a handful of wars, both of my hips were completely shot. The X-rays showed pure bone on bone, with enormous osteophytes. One prominent surgeon said, "You have no choice. Your hips are too far gone; you'll have to have THR." I thought for a moment. Boy, if I'm confused as a physician and sports medicine expert, what chance on earth does the average patient have of making the right decision? One good answer is—because they are both excellent choices! Still, there had to be a right decision.

I began reading the entire world literature. I called doctors in France, England, Belgium, Germany. The more I read, the less I seemed to know. I reached out to Dr. Ronan Treacy, co-inventor of the BHR device, and even the legendary Roger Bannister's son. Both were incredibly thoughtful and helpful. Both said they'd have BHR themselves.

Then I came upon Patricia Walter's Surface Hippy website and read everything on it. Finally, I watched the outstanding Dr. Michael

Mont's video on Pat's website. I went back over my notes and reread the literature, and it suddenly became incredibly clear. What did I really want? I wanted to be able to heli ski, complete the Ironman, ski race, jump out of airplanes, do triathlons, surf bigger waves. I wanted to perform like a 25-year-old again. I had the heart and lungs to do so, but the hips of a 90-year-old. You only live once, so why compromise? Why not go for it? There was the promise of turning back the clock. With Total THR I'd be restricted. Certainly, no surgeon in his right mind would recommend a marathon with a THR. Still, the THR was the safe route. Stick to biking and skiing the groomed slopes, and THR would probably last a lifetime, said one surgeon. THR was a safe bet, a sure bet. The THR operation was faster and the recovery might be quicker as well. But as the star of the hit TV show Dr. Danger, I was expected to do extreme sports, and the THR would never allow that. (Dr. Danger is featured on Amazon Prime.) I spent much of each year in Africa on humanitarian projects (watch featured videos on YouTube called Emergency in Darfur and Sudan: Rising from the Ashes). The decision ended up being a no-brainer. Hip resurfacing with two BHRs.

Here's how I finally made the decision. You'll find that with medical decisions, you're not choosing on the basis of just two key points. There are apt to be many. Also, the decision is not going to be easy. There may be a dozen factors to consider. If you place them side by side and then rate them, you'll come up with a better decision. You're probably not going to make a mistake either way, but there will be differences in how you perform afterward. The most critically important choice is the hospital and surgeon you choose. In medicine, we make a big deal out of what we call outcomes. Simply put, that's how many patients succeed or fail, live or die, have complications or not. I'm a huge believer in the Hospital for Special Surgery in New York City, where I send most patients for joint replacements. It's rated number one in the US for orthopedics. US News & World Report has a good ranking of other national centers of excellence as well as regional centers. Surgeons should be able to provide their actual results for you. This is especially important when operator error plays a big role in poor results. BHR may be the best example. My surgeon had two re-dos out of thousands. The complication rate of 11.6 percent was so high in a published report that many institutions just stopped doing them, and several manufacturers stopped producing the devices.[78] A very good friend had two knees replaced simultaneously. I strongly advised that she go to the Hospital for Special Surgery. Like many patients, she chose convenience over excellence. She saved herself three hours of driving time. One of the knees was installed incorrectly. She had three years of continuing discomfort and pain, and a very long recovery. She saved three hours of driving but sacrificed three years of her life. My advice is to take the time to find the very best and travel to see them. I have many friends from the West Coast who I refer to HSS, and who make the trip.

Simultaneous: I had both of my hips done on the same day. Why? Both needed replacing, and I reckoned that I simply would not know that it was twice as painful. My surgeon, Ed Su, was so good there was no need for transfusions.

My checklist: Here's what my "decision worksheet" for hip surgery looked like. I'd advise you make a similar checklist when you consider surgery and after you have completed extensive homework.

First: I wanted to have a perfect biomechanical result. I'd reviewed this with my boot fitter and ski mechanic, who argued for perfect alignment for ski racing. I could only get that with the BHR.

Second: Yes, there was a higher rate of early failure with the BHR, but it was clear that this was operator dependent. A surgeon just starting out might have a 10 percent failure rate. The great surgeons like Ronan might have a rate of less than one in a thousand. I had great bone quality and thought I'd be pretty compliant as a patient, so I'd have a low risk of fracture, statistically.

Third: I'm so active that I'd need a revision should I live long enough, and the BHR allowed for a much easier revision and a chance to start with a fresh THR femoral implant when the time came. I was

---

78 https://www.ncbi.nlm.nih.gov/pmc/articles/PMC2269024/

at peace with failure, whenever that might be. Down deep, I secretly believed I'd have better longevity with BHR, but without the data.

Fourth: My mother had recently fallen and broken her femur after having had a THR. This caused a type two periprosthetic fracture, which required an open reduction, two plates, screws, wires, etc. This was a far more serious operation, and it took days longer to accomplish than if she had simply fallen and broken her hip. With a BHR, her repair would have been a no-brainer, a simple insertion of the femoral prosthetic device the day of the fracture. THR had put her at much higher risk of a terrible long-term outcome.

Fifth: I clicked the "Athletes Hip Resurfacing Stories" button on the Surface Hippy website. Oh my God!!! An Ironman six months after BHR, I read. That was it. I was determined to do both hips at the same time and be done with it. I'd save five days of hospitalization and five months of rehab, and I'd risk no more complications or blood loss than having one side done.

With the decision made, I needed to find a surgeon. I offered to fly to Birmingham, England, to have one of the inventors do the procedure. There was no need, they graciously said.

"You'll find a Dr. Edwin Su at the Hospital for Special Surgery in New York."

He had their highest recommendation as well as that of every key player I could reach. HSS is considered number one in the US in orthopedics. The hospital's surgeon-in-chief, Tom Sculco, weighed in.

"Ed is one of our very best."

Wow. This was the surgeon my great friend and physiatrist VJ Vad had recommended six months before. I called Dr Su's office on a Friday morning. After fifteen minutes of scrambling, his incredibly effective assistant, Laura Janice, had an operating-room date set for the following Thursday. I had spent the weekend in Aspen boosting my hematocrit up to 48 so I wouldn't need a transfusion. On Monday I had a complete cardiac workup, X-rays, and a visit with Dr. Su. He demonstrated that I had 30-degree hip contractures on both sides.

"Any questions?" he asked.

A month before I would have pummeled him with dozens. I just turned to him and said, "You're the best there is. I just want a near-perfect biomechanical result. You're a great surgeon. and I trust you." The die was cast.

I skied right through my last day before surgery, flew to Washington for a meeting on a young cancer victim in Iraq we were arranging treatment for, and arrived in New York City at 1 a.m. on the day of surgery. I worked out for two hours at the gym, then reported to the hospital. At 1:30 p.m. I was ready for surgery, lying on a gurney with an IV and EKG attached. The curtain opened and Dr. Su appeared.

"I'm psyched," I said.

"So am I," said Dr. Su.

I was wheeled down a long corridor that looked more like a Star Wars bionics laboratory than an OR. Less than four hours later I was in recovery, on my computer, and making a conference call. The following day I walked to the nurse's station and back with crutches. Dr. Su came to visit each morning with a ready smile and an encouraging manner. His bedside manner got a solid A-plus, as did the remarkable team at HSS. I was sad to leave!

By day ten, I had walked a mile on crutches and by day twelve, three miles. Two weeks out, I began to let myself dream of all the things I'd be able to do again that I'd put on hold for so long—a much better pop for surfing, more precise racing turns in skiing, running, rock climbing, even the Ironman. I wondered why I had waited so long. The answer was simple: Most orthopods say that you'll know when you're ready. The truth is that I had been ready for years. While Americans emphasize pain as the main reason for surgery, I had a very high threshold, did tons of yoga, and never had terrible pain. The British emphasize functional criteria. I had a terrible limp, striking waddling gait abnormalities, an abductor lurch, and large hip contractures. As my then-14-year-old son said before surgery, "Dad, you look old, really old." If I had one piece of advice it would be to get a great functional exam and use that to decide rather than deciding based on pain alone. Curiously, all my pain was in my knees. My hips had thrown my biomechanics off so badly that I was at risk of slowly destroying my knees.

Well, I think I've turned back the clock, gained 1.5 inches of height, regained my proper posture, and discovered a miracle that Surface Hippy's Patricia Walter has been a champion of for so long. I've been disappointed by the amount of real expertise and helpful decision-making information on so much of the web. As a physician, I can tell you that website is the best I have ever seen in a medical website. Even now, after my operation, I scroll through the site each evening, picking up new and useful tips on recovery and physical therapy.

When it's time for a replacement

How do you know you have had enough? In the late stages of arthritis, your pain will become harder to control even with injections, and you'll have difficulty sleeping at night. You'll lose a substantial range of motion in your joints, and finally find you are curtailing many of the activities you enjoy. I couldn't walk a full two city blocks in the last stages of my hip arthritis. While you are weighing the risk of an operation, there are two large concerns that loom. First, the loss of mobility may set you up for a severe fall or injury. I was heli-skiing with severe hip arthritis. When I accidentally skied off the edge of a cornice, I braced my fall to protect my painful hips with my right arm and ended up tearing three of the shoulder tendons completely off the bone. The second consideration is that the lack of mobility may lead to weight gain and increased risk factors for diabetes, stroke, and heart disease. Against that background, I'd advise to err on the side of earlier rather than later!

Once you no longer benefit from medications, injections, acupuncture, physical therapy, and braces, the only alternative is to replace the joint. Steroid injections may also hasten the destruction of the joint. Part of the waiting game is to be sure you are old enough that you don't need another joint replacement. As an example, replacing a joint at 40 instead of 60 could mean you'll have to have one or two more joint replacements during your life This is a critically important discussion to have with your orthopedic surgeon. Joint replacements are getting better and better, and their lifespan has increased by a decade or more. Also, there are alternatives such a hip joint resurfacing and partial knee replacement that allow you to have some operative treatment earlier. I've referred several patients in their early forties for hip resurfacing. They were back to horseback riding, surfing, and snowboarding. Should the BHR eventually fail, they still have the chance for a fresh total hip resurfacing. So, for them, there is no need to wait, if their life is truly miserable, and they miss out on all the activities that make life enjoyable. However, since revisions of total hips are difficult, the strategic timing of replacement can help you avoid one. Yes, there is a fine line between too early and too late.

To summarize the disadvantages of waiting too long are as follows:

Loss of mobility

Increased risk of falls

Increased risk of chronic illness

Difficulty of full rehabilitation once too much muscle and fitness has been lost

Too Early: Many responsible orthopedists will turn you away if there is still much to be gained by non-surgical therapy. I wrote an entire book about this called Wear and Tear: Stop the Pain and Put the Spring Back in Your Body. For instance, joint mobility can be vastly improved with a concentrated period of yoga. Joint injections can also extend usage, though you risk joint damage. For knees, improving quad strength and losing weight decreases pain. You may also lack the motivation to undergo the arduous rehabilitation required to fully recover and end up with long loss of mobility.

Outcomes: In choosing the right surgeon, you of course want superb credentials, experience, and reputation. However, a big piece of low complications and high success is in great anesthesiology and support staff and low infection and readmission rates for the hospital. In picking a surgeon and hospital, look for terrific outcomes. You want a surgeon who specializes in just one joint, has low mobility complications, and has a very low infection rate. US News & World Report gives you a good rough cut on the best orthopedic hospitals since they have the systems in place to get terrific results.

HSS also performs more hip and knee replacements than any other US hospital and is ranked the number-one hospital for orthopedics in the United States by U.S. News & World Report. No other hospital in the world focuses solely on health problems of the bones, joints, and soft tissues like muscles. This is where I had my hips resurfaced and where I send my own patients and family.

The success rate for hip replacement surgery at HSS is very high. In a study, HSS interviewed patients to learn about their progress. Two years after their surgeries, 99.4 percent of patients said they had relief from pain, 98.8 percent said their ability to move was improved, and 97.8 percent said their quality of life was better because of their surgery. (Source: HSS Arthroplasty Registry, 2007-2012.)

Ankle: Severe arthritis of the ankle joint is the result of progressive wearing down of the articular cartilage cushion that lines the joint, ultimately resulting in bone-on-bone grinding of the joint surface. Fusion has been the procedure of choice. The alternative is a total ankle replacement, coming into widespread use in the late Nineties. Forgoing the fusion process, this procedure instead relies on replacement of the arthritic surfaces with a man-made implant that is composed of two or three components that glide against each other, using low-friction materials. The primary benefit is pain relief with retained ankle motion. I have a patient in her mid-thirties and have recommended this operation. There are no long-term results of more than ten years.

There are several advantages over a fusion:

Less joint stress, so less risk of arthritis
Back in action faster
Much greater function, with range of motion much improved

Knee replacement

When you need knee replacement surgery: As physical therapy, anti-inflammatory medication, injections, and weight loss no longer provide relief, have a surgical evaluation. Other key signs you may need surgery are these:

Knees are stiff and swollen
Pain throughout the day, even at rest
Great difficulty walking, getting out of a chair, or climbing or
    descending stairs

Total knee replacement: The majority of patients who need to have their entire joint replaced have suffered severe damage to the cartilage that cushions the knee joint, often due to arthritis, injury, and continued wear and tear. Surgeons replace the damaged cartilage with metal or plastic replacements that restore the smooth gliding function of your knees and eliminate the pain.

Partial knee replacement: If you're fortunate, you may have damaged only one compartment of the knee, perhaps due to an old sports injury. In this case, you'll enjoy great relief of pain and an increase in mobility by just replacing one compartment of your knee.

Same-day knee replacement: Incredibly, some patients may go home the same day as the procedure if they're in good health, don't smoke, and have a great support team at home. You'll benefit from a lower risk of infection and a faster return to normal activities while enjoying your recovery at home. The operation lasts one to one and a half hours.

How long it will last: The life expectancy of the newer-technology knee replacements are astounding, lasting fifteen to twenty years in most patients. Other advancements include smaller incisions and regional anesthesia, which isolates the area around the knee.

Rehabilitation: Much of the structural strength of the knee joint is due to the muscles that cause it to flex, contract, and stabilize.

Maintaining these as long as possible before surgery will ensure a quicker and more effective rehabilitation. After surgery, it's vital to regain your strength and mobility for the replacement to be fully effective.

Hip replacement

When to replace your hips: Consider surgery when you suffer severe pain that limits sleep, work, and the enjoyment of everyday activities, and anti-inflammatory pain relievers no longer control the pain. Be careful not to let the pain get so severe that you are offered opioids. Surgery is nearly always preferable to starting opioids, with all the risks, complications and side effects they have.

Restricted joint range of motion that makes walking and other activities of daily living difficult is a key indication you could benefit from surgery. I could barely walk a block and half before my hip surgery.

Kinds of hip surgery

Birmingham Hip Resurfacing (BHR): This is the operation that changed my life. The BHR is especially appealing for very young patients. I have referred some in their early forties for whom a total hip replacement was not recommended. There is an upper age limit of roughly 60 for BHR for females, with the smaller size of the ball of their hip joint and a higher risk of complication. Also, very few orthopedic surgeons do these, and even fewer get great results. I highly recommend my own surgeon, Edwin Su at HSS.

Total hip replacement (THR): This is the more common operation and is just getting better and better, with less pain and faster mobilization after surgery. Your surgeon will replace the socket with a durable plastic cup and your femoral head with a ceramic or metal alloy ball. The ball sits on a metal step which is inserted down the middle of your femur.

Risks of hip replacement

Infection: Infection is number one. You want to ask your hospital and surgeon what their surgical infection rate is.

HSS is a leader in preventing infection. The New York Department of Health reports that out of more than 160 hospitals in New York that did hip replacements in 2014, only HSS had a hip replacement surgery site infection (SSI) rate that was "significantly lower than the state average" for that year, and that those infection rates at HSS had been significantly lower than the state average in each of the seven years between 2008–2014.

Blood clots: Accidental dislocation in recovery. Be careful! This is the one time in life when doctors say you should take it easy ... and you really should to let your new hip set.

How long hip implants last: Technology has made tremendous strides in the survival of hip implants. The general figure is ten to twenty years, but some patients are getting even more years out of them. Your age and the type of implant you choose affects the implant's longevity. A 2008 study of more than 50,000 patients who had THR surgery at age 55 or older reported that between 71 percent and 94 percent still had well-working implants after fifteen years.[79] This too is where the risk-benefit equation comes in. If you are 60, you'll likely need a replacement at 80, when you may be weaker and have a harder time recovering. Replace at 70, and you may get to 90. Offsetting this, though, is the years of enjoyment you may sacrifice, and the fitness you'd attain with earlier surgery. Re-do operations are often not as good as the original, so you'll want a top center of excellence to operate.

When can I drive: The safe guideline is to wait six weeks. I flew my airplane a week after my implants and drove the same day ... cautiously.

---

79 (Source: Makela, Keijo T. MD; Eskelinen, Antti, et al. "Total Hip Arthroplasty for Primary Osteoarthritis in Patients Fifty-five Years of Age or Older: An Analysis of the Finnish Arthroplasty Registry." Journal of Bone & Joint Surgery – American Volume – Vol 90 October 01, 2008.)

What about metal detectors: This is a big "yes." You'll send TSA scrambling. Always ask for the body scanners, which are a godsend to patients with joint replacements, since you won't have to be patted down. They're in nearly every airport.

Simultaneous replacement of left and right hips: Yes!!! If arthritis is responsible for your hip pain and disability, chances are that both hips will need to be replaced. I opted to do both at the same time. My philosophy was you wouldn't know how much more two hurt than one—just do it! You'll need to be in good health and 75 or younger.

Coda

Failure!!! So, after all my extraordinary efforts in training, nutrition, and lifestyle it appeared as if I had lost the big game of life. The program just had not worked. Aging had won. Just a giant waste of time. Why? My CT angiogram, a picture of the arteries in my heart, showed massive amounts of calcium. "Finished," I mused. I talked to my family about my will. The radiologist reading concluded that I had severe coronary artery disease. The British Columbia study we looked at had concluded that 10 percent of Master athletes had severe coronary artery disease, and I was certainly one of them. I called a classmate of mine, Karl Krieger, MD, a senior cardiovascular surgeon at New York-Presbyterian, where I referred many patients.

"Have a cath," Karl recommended.

A "cath" is jargon for a cardiac cauterization, where a long hollow tube is threaded directly into the coronary arteries to determine the degree of blockage.

"Caths are so low-risk now, and if you have a real problem, you'll find it and fix it."

My cardiologist, Dartmouth-Hitchcock's Jon Wahrenberger, agreed. I had planned to go to MGH or the Cleveland Clinic, where I referred most of my patients' friends and family.

"Our Jimmy DeVries is someone I'd send my own family to," Jon said.

Jimmy was Dartmouth-Hitchcock's lead interventional cardiologist. After a wistful drive down to DHMC and some blood work, the nurses rolled me into the main angiogram room. Jimmy proved to be a fun, relaxed, and extremely competent cardiologist.

"Would you like a sedative?" he asked.

"No thanks! Wouldn't miss this for the world."

Jimmy skillfully threaded a narrow tube through my radial artery and up into my heart. My coronary arteries appeared on a huge TV screen as Jimmy shot dye into them to examine each artery individually for blockages. Given the CT angiogram results, a noninvasive test that lights up coronary arteries and outlines blockages with a special contrast agent, we all expected to find substantial disease and were already planning how stents might be placed in the most severe blockages. We even talked about bypass surgery, should there be too many blockages. After a suspenseful few minutes, the screen displayed a blockage right in the left anterior descending artery, a blockage called a widow-maker. Should he place a stent? Was it risky and in danger of breaking and clotting off the artery, causing a heart attack? So, you can just imagine what it feels like to like on a table with a tube stuck right into the most vital and dangerous part of your heart, waiting to see what might happen! A sudden arrhythmia? Crushing chest pain from a piece of plaque broken loose? Before the procedure, the cardiologist had warned that the complications were piercing the artery, stroke, or death. To determine how dangerous the blockage was, Jimmy then performed a technique called iFR (instant flow reserve), which measures the pressure before and after the blockage. Jon came into the room to weigh in as the results appeared on the screen. If the readings were 1.0 at the top before the blockage and 0.5 at the bottom, there would be a big problem with vastly reduced pressure and blood flow, and Jimmy would likely place a wire mesh stent to open the artery and keep it open. Then the results of the pressure test popped up open the screen ... 0.91! Nearly perfect blood flow! Then Jimmy looked at the rest of my arteries. Like pieces of fine art, they were big, bouncy, elastic, and full of life, with hundreds of fine small vessels all perfectly formed. I had won!!!

The cardiologists said, "We never see coronary arteries like these!"

All those years of training had paid off. I showed Jimmy my WHOOP scores, with HRVs averaging 70. I had reset the youth switch to that of a teenager, and now I had the coronary arteries to prove it. What accounted for all the calcium on the calcium scan? Jimmy told me that the heart had good and bad remodeling. On the inside of the arteries all the remodeling led to blockages, heart disease, and risk of a heart attack and death. On the outside, the calcium remodeling could be considered healthy remodeling from the stresses of aging and life. This healthy outside remodeling is what I had. That remodeling is what the calcium scan test was picking up—without the ability to discern which was good or bad. Jon then walked in the recovery room with my latest LDL cholesterol level. 65! Just where the Cleveland Clinic's famous Steve Nissen, MD, wanted it. I drove home that evening just delighted. I had won. My coronaries looked like they were good for another twenty years. I'd flipped the youth switch. Gratitude washed over me. Grateful to Dartmouth-Hitchcock, John, and Jimmy. Just a fabulous medical center and a great team. Grateful for the support of my family.

So, as a physician and a patient, I'd just like to conclude by saying, this journey is the most important you'll ever undertake, and the most worthwhile and satisfying of all. Don't approach risk factors and illness with fear and trepidation. Approach them like a warrior prepared to confront and vanquish your demons. You can fully flip the youth switch and battle the demons of chronic illness to become one of life's big winners. Good luck. You're going to crush it!!!

APPENDIX:

RESOURCES

GEAR: WEARABLE TECH

You'll discover the greatest training and fitness revolutions in wearable technology. These jewel-like devices will transform your workout, making them both far more precise and efficient while easier and more enjoyable, allowing you to crush it. There are excellent sites such as DC Rainmaker that have fabulous reviews on all the devices. I'm a careful buyer, read the reviews, try all the devices, and carefully test them. What I have listed below are the devices I have found work the best and provide the most useful information. These are ones I have paid full retail price for and have given no endorsements.

Garmin Forerunner

Any of the Forerunner series are terrific and range from as little as $75 to over $500. You can still key data even with the much less expensive devices.

Garmin Forerunner 945 GPS

This is the new Rolls Royce of training devices. I record every workout every day with this. There are highly specialized settings for sports like SUP where I can review my stroke rate and even which distance my stroke takes me. This automatically downloads to my iPhone, my Garmin desktop, the Training Peaks app, and my coach. I always wear a chest strap for the heart rate monitor because the wrist heart rates tend to over-exaggerate the intensity of a workout.

Pros: It's robust. It works forever. It includes most major sports, including SUP, with special settings for stroke cadence and length. It interfaces with the most exotic gear from SmO2 to power meters. It's important to use a chest strap for heart rate, or you'll get erratic recordings during training if you rely on the wrist.

Cons: Menus are difficult and don't make much sense. For instance, even if you have used it for years, the first menu choice presents a new watch face rather than changing sensors or training programs. Also, they love to make it beep! It inexplicably goes black and beeps every 15 minutes or so during training, and it beeps all day and night for email and messages. If you turn "do not disturb" on, the device turns it off a few hours later! Nonetheless, it's my first choice. It even records pulse oxygen.

The Garmin App

Pros: The app stores and displays all the training data you have recorded on your Garmin Forerunner. It has nice geographical maps and graphic display of all values.

Cons: It doesn't scale the data, so it's sometimes hard to discern. As an example, SmO2 data might range from 69-75, but Garmin will show you 0-100. Garmin doesn't have any apparent AI to make sense out of the data. Even if you're a serious athlete, it keeps congratulating you for the number of steps you've taken each day. Steps are not a metric any serious athlete I know values!

WHOOP

There is no better way of knowing when you are ready to hammer and when you need to recover than WHOOP. The AI insights are the most advanced of any platform. It records every heartbeat as a sophisticated EKG, plus sleep metrics and strain.

Pros: Fantastic use of graphics and design. It has very well thought out AI for sleep and recovery, and now also prescribes the amount of strain you can benefit from each day.

Cons: You can't see real-time scores. It doesn't give you on actual HRV figure on the iPhone app. While the wrist HR is good, it doesn't rival chest HR for accuracy, so strain scores may be a bit off. Still, it's my favorite platform of all and ever improving.

SmO2

Simply the best way to measure exercise intensity and recovery during a workout.

Humon Hex: This is super easy to put on and use, and it has a color-coded system for intensities that I use for all my intervals. My favorite technique for determining threshold muscle oxygen consumption uses an SmO2 device. The Humon turns orange as you approach threshold. Place it on the biggest muscle group you'll use during your sport. For instance, I'll put it right on the quad for cycling, Nordic skiing, hill bounding, and SUP. When the Humon hits red, you've really overdone it and can't expect to continue at that pace for long. However, this is great for interval training, since you will know if you're going hard enough. If the Humon is not turning red, you're not going hard enough. Love the ability of measuring real-time human physiology rather than relying on approximations based on age and heart rate.

Cons: Sometimes it's hard to interface with Garmin.

Moxy: This gives you a larger range of SmO2 readings and claims higher accuracy.

Cons: It has a really messy tape system for attaching and a higher cost.

Heart rate chest strap

This is vital to getting accurate heart rates. None of the wrist-based devices are accurate enough during a workout to be helpful. Garmin makes inexpensive and long-lasting straps available on Amazon. Cheap!

Apple Watch

The primary benefit of the Apple Watch is detecting abnormal heart rates, specifically atrial fibrillation. Apple doesn't yet have sophisticated AI or training software.

Pros: It detects atrial fibrillation.

Cons: It's impossible to set up. It took me over a week, and I still couldn't figure it out!

Waterproof iPod Shuffle

Love these for the 32-mile Molokai 2 Oahu race and 50K Nordic ski races! It uses a waterproof iPod Mini and super-lightweight waterproof earphones. I create playlists on iTunes and transfer them for each race to coincide with various challenges. For example, at the four-hour mark, I put my boldest rock music on for the churning seas off of Koko Head near the end of Molokai 2 Oahu. I recommend the Hydroharmony headphones, since they stay put. I have had so many audio mishaps racing with earphone buds, which become dislodged so easily. These Hydroharmonies have a solid piece of lightweight plastic that holds the earphones in place.

Delphin

The Delphin was made for those who prefer streaming audio, and it works with Spotify, Pandora, Audible, Apple Music, Amazon Music, Soundcloud, and Podcast and Radio Addict.

Problems solved: Ultra-lightweight waterproof performance audio that doesn't come off during even the toughest competition. **Cool feature:** It weighs little more than a quarter! www.underwateraudio.com/collections waterproof-headphones

Technology Training Platforms

Online training platforms now do most of the work of coaching for you. Here's a brief look:

WHOOP

This most ingenious of training platforms uses artificial intelligence based on your data and the data of many other athletes like you to determine what your training load should be like for the day. If you have a bright green high-recovery day, you'll be asked for a high training load. I reviewed the platform with Emily Capodilupo, WHOOP's resident AI guru, and it is pure genius.

Training Peaks

Most coaches use this platform to deliver your daily training program and follow your progress. I love the training stress chart best; it shows your overall training load, fatigue, and form factors. I rely on this to taper for races. TP uses the most sophisticated formula to determine training zones.

Garmin

This tracks the most important variables, and I review my data every day. For instance, for SUP I can see:

Speed
Heart rate
Distance

Stroke rate

Stroke cadence

Muscle oxygen consumption

There are nice graphing functions, though it's surprising that they don't do a better job of autoscaling. (See above.) The platform itself has no discernible intelligence or AI, so it won't help you plan workouts or learn from them, as WHOOP does.

SLEEP GEAR

Melatonin, Nature Made Adult Gummies

Bose noise-cancelling earphones

Bose sleep buds: They can generate white noise, ocean, rain forest, etc.

Tart cherry juice before sleep

Eye masks

Tempur-Pedic pillows

Blue light-blocking glasses: Use this site to be sure that yours work! Look through your glasses at the picture on the site and you can see if they work! (blueblockglasses.com/blogs/news/the-rgb-color-model-test-how-effective-is-your-blue-light-filter-eyewear)

SPORTS QUIVERS

"Sports quivers" are specialized equipment for your favorite sport. For improved performance and far greater comfort, I have specialized gear for each sport, which I call my quiver!

Cycling road bike: Carbon fiber Serotta with lightweight wheels; it's a super-light bike with phenomenal acceleration due to carbon fiber wheel set and tubular tires.

Cycling time-trial bike: Cervelo P5 with electric gear shifting
Cycling uphill racing mountain bike: Carbon fiber Santa Cruz

Skimo: Pierre Gignoux custom carbon fiber racing boots—the single finest piece of exercise gear I have. Allows for stunning downhill performance with the lightest weight of any boot.

Dynafit parka and pants

Skitrab Gara Aero Sprint: The fastest ski uphill and surprisingly great downhill. I ski it every morning up Perry Merrill in Stowe.

Skitrab Ski Gara Aero World Cup 70 19/20 (Size 171): Long, stiff Skimo race ski that allows greater stability and speeds.

Salomon Minim race ski

SUP:
SIC Maui Custom 20.5 inch, 14-foot race board
SIC Maui Standamaran: Ideal for the messy waters of the Carolina
    Cup; I have two of these
SIC Maui Bayonet 17-foot Downwind board
SIC Maui Bayonet V3 custom race board
King Paddle Sports 19-foot flat water race board
Speedboard 19-foot race board
Starboard 18-foot Ace Downwind
Starboard 14-foot Ace Downwind
Starboard 14-foot x 23-inch Sprint

Nordic:
Salomon Waxless Classic race skis
Fischer Double Poling Classic skis
Fischer Classic and Skate race skis
Salomon Classic race boots
Pierre Gignoux custom skate boots
Swix 3.0 race poles

CARDIAC RISK

www.aafp.org/afp/2010/0801/p265.html
www.cardiosmart.org/Tools/Heart-Disease-Risk-Assessment